Handbook for Dental Nurses

Handbook for Dental Nurses

Jane A. Bonehill
Clare L. Roberts
Diana R. Wincott

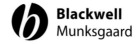

Blackwell
Munksgaard

© 2007 by Jane A. Bonehill, Clare L. Roberts and Diana R. Wincott

Blackwell Publishing editorial offices:
Blackwell Publishing Ltd, 9600 Garsington Road, Oxford OX4 2DQ, UK
    Tel: +44 (0)1865 776868
Blackwell Publishing Professional, 2121 State Avenue, Ames, Iowa
50014-8300, USA
    Tel: +1 515 292 0140
Blackwell Publishing Asia Pty Ltd, 550 Swanston Street, Carlton,
Victoria 3053, Australia
    Tel: +61 (0)3 8359 1011

The right of the Author to be identified as the Author of this Work has
been asserted in accordance with the Copyright, Designs and Patents
Act 1988.

First published 2007 by Blackwell Publishing Ltd

ISBN: 978-1-4051-2803-2

Library of Congress Cataloging-in-Publication Data
Bonehill, Jane A.
    Handbook for dental nurses / Jane A. Bonehill, Clare L. Roberts,
    Diana R. Wincott.
            p.   ;   cm.
    Includes bibliographical references and index.
    ISBN: 978-1-4051-2803-2 (pbk. : alk. paper)
    1. Dental assistants—Handbooks, manuals, etc.   I. Roberts,
    Clare L.   II. Wincott, Diana R.   III. Title.
    [DNLM: 1. Dental Assistants—Handbooks.   2. Dental Care—
    methods—Handbooks.   WU 90 B712h 2007]

    RK60.5.B467 2007
    617.6′0233—dc22   2006100269

A catalogue record for this title is available from the British Library

Set in 9/11 pt Palatino by SNP Best-set Typesetter Ltd., Hong Kong
Printed and bound in Singapore by Markono Print Media Pte Ltd

The publisher's policy is to use permanent paper from mills that
operate a sustainable forestry policy, and which has been manufactured
from pulp processed using acid-free and elementary chlorine-free
practices. Furthermore, the publisher ensures that the text paper and
cover board used have met acceptable environmental accreditation
standards.

For further information on Blackwell Publishing, visit our website:
www.blackwellmunksgaard.com

Contents

Preface

As three experienced dental nurses, we understand how difficult it is to retain all the knowledge you learnt during training while also keeping up to date with developments in dentistry. Our aim is to provide a practical, quick reference handbook, which is easy to understand, and helps dental nurses to maintain high standards in clinical practice.

This is not an academic text. We do not recommend that you read the book from cover to cover. It would be better to read chunks of the book when you need information on a particular topic.

The focus is on checklists, helpful hints and practical information. Photographs and diagrams help show good practice in all aspects of dental nursing. We have also included guidance on: how to improve your working life, maintaining health and wellbeing, raising awareness of the implications of new legislation, the importance of team working and some ideas on future career options, including continuing professional development.

We hope that the book will:

(1) Give user friendly information to help newly qualified dental nurses who want to check key facts and confirm that they have not forgotten anything important.
(2) Update and support dental nurse returners during their transition back to work.
(3) Be a useful addition to the practice library as an induction tool and reference for all the team.
(4) Assist 'grandparented' dental nurses and encourage them to continue learning and improving their chairside skills.

Who would benefit from reading this book?

- Newly qualified dental nurses
- Returners
- Grandparented dental nurses
- Assessors and trainers
- New staff

We would like to thank:

A very dear friend Toni Kelly who proof read some of the chapters.

Eileen Layhe for her expertise on implants.

Sharon Iommi and Shakespeare Drive Dental Centre for allowing us to take photographs.

Richard Clifford, Pat Johnson and Alison Ofield.

Colleagues who are too numerous to mention for their support throughout the writing of this book.

Author profiles

Jane A. Bonehill

Jane has been a member of the dental team for almost 30 years and has a wide experience in dental nursing, reception and practice management. She is the proprietor of DenMed Training and Consultancy and works with dental companies around the UK, delivering certificated training courses and providing consultancy to assist dental teams in the management of health and safety.

Jane is an active member of the British Association of Dental Nurses and holds office on the Health and Safety Advisory Committee. She is a Technician Safety Practitioner with the Institution of Occupational Health and Safety and a Licentiate Member of the Chartered Institute of Personnel and Development.

Since 2001, Jane has been a part time External Verifier for City & Guilds and is currently studying for their Mentoring Award.

Clare L. Roberts

Clare has been dental nursing for 18 years; she worked in general dental practice before training at Guy's Dental Hospital. Clare is currently Research and Development Manager at Guy's, Kings and St Thomas' Dental Nurse Education and Training Centre. She has been awarded a grant by Colgate for DCP research. Clare is responsible for designing, delivering and managing new training initiatives at the centre. She is an active member of the British Association of Dental Nurses and has chaired their National Teaching Group and Health & Safety Advisory Committee. Clare is a member of the National Examining Board for Dental Nurses

Panel of Examiners and has recently been appointed as a General Dental Council (GDC) Inspector of Dental Care Professionals courses and examinations.

Clare has already written a distance learning programme.

Diana R. Wincott MBE

Diana has been involved in dental nursing for over 40 years, first in general dental practice and then in four London dental teaching hospitals. Diana has played an influential part in promoting dental nurses and has served as President of the British Association of Dental Nurses and in 1995 became the first dental nurse to be elected as the Chairman of the National Examining Board for Dental Nurses. Since 1979, Diana has worked with the General Dental Council firstly on the Dental Nurses Standards and Training Board drawing up training objectives for Dental Nurses and more recently as a member of the PCD Curricula Overview Group. Diana has recently been appointed as a GDC Inspector of Dental Care Professionals courses and examinations, and as a Director of the National Examining Board for Dental Nurses.

Diana was awarded an MBE in 1998 for services to dentistry.

Daily Routine Maintenance

1

Systematic start of day preparation and correct
end of the day close down of the clinical
environment is essential so that the dental team
can work efficiently. It ensures the control of
infection, and the safety and security of the
dental establishment.

START OF DAY SURGERY SET UP

On arrival
- Arrive at least 15 minutes prior to the first patient
  appointment.
- Change into surgery attire (clinical 'uniform' should not be
  worn outside the practice).
- Switch on all power sources – lighting, air-conditioning (if
  applicable, if not open a window) air compressor, suction
  unit, dental chair, autoclave, dental unit and computer (if
  applicable).

Test autoclave
- Wipe door seals, fill up water reservoir (check with manufacturer's guidelines for water type), place process indicator strip
  on tray, close the door and start a normal cycle (check with
  manufacturer's guidelines if this should be with or without a
  load).
- Record the following details* (if the autoclave has a recorder
  or printer examine the record for compliance) (Figure 1.1):
  –date, time, serial number and location of unit;
  –cycle counter number;

1. Serial number:		2. Location:		
3. Date:		4. Time:		

ACTIVITY	ITEM	EVIDENCE		COMMENTS OR ACTION
(1)	Cycle counter number			
(2)	Time to reach holding temperature			
(3)	Temperature during holding period*			
(4)	Pressure during holding period*			
(5)	Total time at holding temperature			
(6)	Water drained at end of previous day	YES	NO	
(7)	Initial of authorised user			
(8)	Door seals secure	YES	NO	
(9)	Door safety devices functioning correctly	YES	NO	
(10)	Any comments:			
(11)	Name of Tester	Signature of Tester		

*Only applicable if autoclave has temperature/pressure displays/gauges.
Please attach each Time, Steam and Temperature TST strip to this test sheet.
Additional comments:

Fig. 1.1 Daily autoclave test sheet.

  –time to reach holding temperature;
  –temperature during holding period*;
  –pressure during holding period*;
  –total time at holding temperature/pressure;
  –water drained at end of previous day;
  –initials of authorised user;
  –door seals secure;
  –door safety devices functioning correctly;
  –any comments;
  –name of tester.

*Only applicable if autoclave has temperature/pressure displays/gauges

If the following conditions are achieved the autoclave can be used:

- 'cycle complete' signal is visible;
- record shows cycle temperatures and pressures are within expected range;
- door could not be operated until 'cycle complete' signal is visible;
- no abnormalities.

Surgery set-up (Figure 1.2)
(1) Test operating light, X-ray switch and arm.
(2) Put on heavy-duty protective gloves, mask, safety goggles and plastic apron.
(3) Fill up the ultrasonic bath with appropriate solution.
(4) Fill up the 'cold disinfectant' reservoir.
(5) Clear handpiece tubes and 3-in-1 syringe by running water through them.
(6) Fill up the water bottle and attach to unit, run water through (check manufacturer's guidelines for recommended time)
(7) Disinfect and wipe all surfaces and equipment.
(8) Place operating chair at appropriate level.
(9) Remove heavy-duty protective gloves, mask and safety goggles.
(10) Cover light handles, all handpieces on dental unit and suction unit and tubing, switches, control panels, and headrest on chair with disposable plastic sheaths/covers.
(11) Check appointment schedule and ensure laboratory items are available.
(12) Set up instrument treatment tray for first patient and ensure this remains covered until patient is seated.
(13) Place personal protective equipment/clothing (PPE/C) in appropriate position for dental personnel and patient.
(14) Make available all dental records relating to first patient.

END OF DAY SURGERY CLOSE DOWN (Figure 1.3)
(1) Put on heavy-duty protective gloves, mask, safety goggles and plastic apron:

DATE: Day.............................. Month.............................. Year..............................

SURGERY NAME/NUMBER:..............................

TASK	DONE ✓	INITIAL	COMMENTS
(1) Switch on power sources			
(2) Ventilate surgery (open window)			
(3) Fill up autoclave water reservoir			
(4) Wipe autoclave door seals			
(5) Carry out autoclave test cycle			
(6) Test operating light			
(7) Test x-ray switch and arm			
(8) Fill ultrasonic bath			
(9) Fill up 'cold disinfectant' reservoir			
(10) Flush through handpiece and 3-in-1 tubes			
(11) Fill dental unit water bottle and run water through			

(12) Disinfect surfaces and equipment					
(13) Place operating light at appropriate level					
(14) Place operating chair at appropriate level					
(15) Place disposable sheaths on equipment					
(16) Check appointment schedule for laboratory items					
(17) Set up instrument tray and keep covered					
(18) Personal protective equipment/clothing placed ready for use					
(19) Dental records placed ready for use					

Complete the checklist at the START of every day in each clinical area/surgery. The checklist should be retained for a period determined by the policy of your practice.

DETAILS OF PERSON COMPLETING THIS FORM

NAME: **SIGNATURE:**   **DATE:**

Fig. 1.2 Start of day surgery set-up checklist. Please apply the above as is appropriate for your practice; some of the tasks may not be appropriate for all surgeries.

DATE: Day................................... Month.............................. Year...............

SURGERY NAME/NUMBER:.......................

TASK	DONE ✓	INITIAL	COMMENTS
(1) Disinfect work surfaces			
(2) Disinfect surgery equipment			
(3) Remove disposable sheaths			
(4) Flush suction lines through			
(5) Empty dental unit water bottle, leave to dry			
(6) Empty 'cold disinfectant' reservoir, leave to dry			
(7) Empty ultrasonic bath, rinse and dry			
(8) Empty autoclave, transfer instruments to storage area			
(9) Dry autoclave chamber, leave door ajar			
(10) Clean sinks			

(11) Empty clinical bins and replace sacks					
(12) Raise dental chair to highest position					
(13) Clear all work surfaces					
(14) Restock consumables					
(15) Close windows and adjust heating levels					
(16) Switch off water supply					
(17) Switch off power sources					
(18) Return dental records to storage area					
(19) Take clinical waste to storage area					

Complete the checklist at the **END** of every day in each clinical area/surgery. The checklist should be retained for a period determined by the policy of the practice.

DETAILS OF PERSON COMPLETING THIS FORM

NAME: **SIGNATURE:**   **DATE:**

Fig. 1.3 End of day surgery close down checklist. Please apply the above as it is appropriate for your practice; some of the tasks may not be appropriate for all surgeries.

(a) decontaminate work surfaces and surgery equipment and carry out decontamination of dental instruments as described in Chapter 2;

(b) remove disposable sheaths from all equipment;

(c) flush suction lines through according to manufacturer's instructions;

(d) empty water bottle on unit, rinse and leave to dry;

(e) empty 'cold disinfectant' reservoir and leave to dry;

(f) empty solution from ultrasonic bath, rinse and dry;

(g) drain autoclave of water, dry the chamber and leave door slightly open;

(h) clean sinks with soapy water, rinse and spray with recommended substance;

(i) empty clinical waste bins and replace with new sacks;

(j) remove personal protective equipment and clothing (PPE/C).

(2) Raise chair for easy cleaning underneath.

(3) Ensure all work surfaces are clear.

(4) Replace consumables where necessary in order to optimise stock levels.

(5) Close windows and adjust heating levels.

(6) Switch off water supply and all power sources including lights.

(7) Return patient records to secure area.

(8) Remove clinical waste sacks and take to waste store.

(9) Change out of 'clinical uniform' before leaving the dental environment.

TOP TIPS

1. Use a 'Start of day surgery set up' and 'End of day surgery close down checklist'; tick each task when you have completed it and sign to confirm; you can also make any relevant comments relating to each task (Figures 1.2 and 1.3).

2. Use the above checklist as an induction aide-memoire for new nurses.

3. Do not leave the autoclave in operation at the end of the day, if time is limited contaminated instruments should be left on a tray clearly marked 'NON STERILE'.
4. If you identify any faults with items of equipment or instruments report it immediately to the designated person.
5. Always refer to manufacturer's guidelines relating to equipment, instruments and chemical solutions.
6. Check policy for disposal of substances; it may not be permissible to empty contaminated water and disinfectants in the sink.
7. Remove PPE/C before leaving the clinical area.

LINKS TO OTHER CHAPTERS
- Chapter 2 – Control of Infection.
- Chapter 16 – Health and Safety in the Dental Environment.

FURTHER READING
Prestige Medical Autoclaving Fact Sheet No 4. Prestige, April 2006.

Infection Control

> Cross-infection control procedures must
> be carried out to the highest possible
> standard to ensure the protection of
> patients and the dental team.

Dental nurses have both ethical and legal responsibilities to control the spread of infection. This is most effectively achieved through adopting universal precautions.

UNIVERSAL PRECAUTIONS
(Hazardous Waste Regulations 2005 may affect the principle of universal precautions due to the 'new' definitions and classifications of healthcare waste (see Chapter 16).)

In simple terms this is defined as: 'the same routine high standards of cross-infection control are carried out for all patients and all dental treatments'. Universal precautions should be applied throughout the following ten key areas to reduce the risk of the spread of infection:

(1) Personal hygiene
(2) Personal protective clothing/equipment (PPE/C)
(3) Clinical procedures
(4) Environment
(5) Decontamination of equipment and surfaces
(6) Decontamination of instruments
(7) Waste disposal
(8) Immunisation
(9) Laboratory procedures
(10) Training

(1) When washing hands apply quantity of product to wet hands.

When disinfecting hands apply recommended quantity to dry hands

(5) Backs of fingers to opposing palms with fingers interlocked, concentrate on the fingertips

(2) Palm to palm

(6) Rotational rubbing of right thumb clasped in left palm and vice versa

(3) Right palm over left dorsum and left palm over right dorsum

(7) Rotational rubbing, backwards and forwards with clasped fingers of right hand in left palm and vice versa

(4) Palm to palm and fingers interlocked

(8) Rotational rubbing of right wrist clasped in left palm and vice versa

Fig. 2.1 Hand hygiene technique. (Reproduced with permission of Schulke and Mayr UK Ltd, Sheffield, 2004.)

Dental nurses should use the following guidelines to ensure they are carrying out their ethical and legal responsibilities.

PERSONAL HYGIENE

To prevent the spread of infection through inter-personal contact.

❏ Hands washed prior to touching equipment, surfaces, instruments.
❏ Hands washed using the Ayliffe, Babb and Quoraishi method (Figure 2.1).
❏ Hands washed using skin disinfectant.

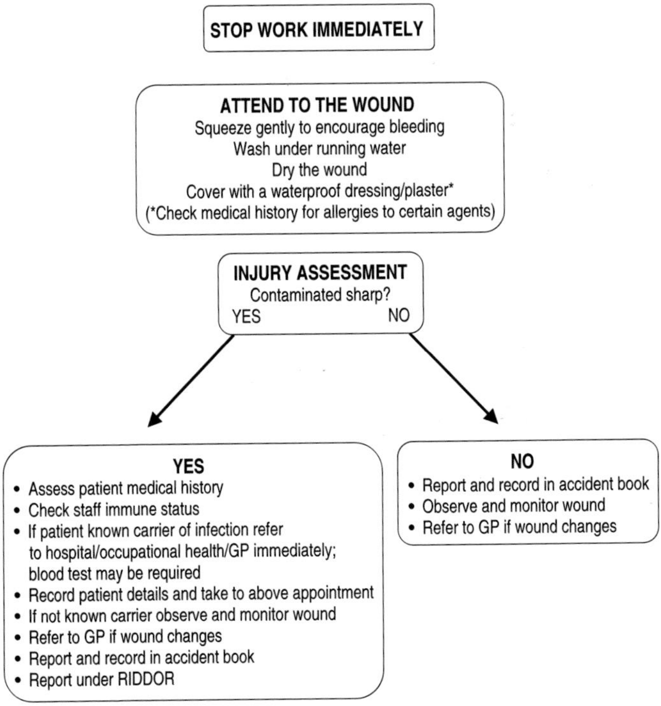

STOP WORK IMMEDIATELY

ATTEND TO THE WOUND
Squeeze gently to encourage bleeding
Wash under running water
Dry the wound
Cover with a waterproof dressing/plaster*
(*Check medical history for allergies to certain agents)

INJURY ASSESSMENT
Contaminated sharp?
YES   NO

YES
- Assess patient medical history
- Check staff immune status
- If patient known carrier of infection refer
  to hospital/occupational health/GP immediately;
  blood test may be required
- Record patient details and take to above appointment
- If not known carrier observe and monitor wound
- Refer to GP if wound changes
- Report and record in accident book
- Report under RIDDOR

NO
- Report and record in accident book
- Observe and monitor wound
- Refer to GP if wound changes

Fig. 2.2 Procedure followed after a sharps injury.

❏ Hand creams applied at end of session.
❏ Cuts and abrasions covered.
❏ Take immediate action in the event of inoculation (sharps) injuries (Figure 2.2).
❏ Rings, wrist watches, visible body jewellery (excluding stud earrings) and bracelets removed prior to beginning work.
❏ Nail polish removed, nails are clean and short.
❏ Clinical uniform changed daily or when visibly contaminated.
❏ Clinical uniform is worn only in the practice.
❏ Footwear is clean.

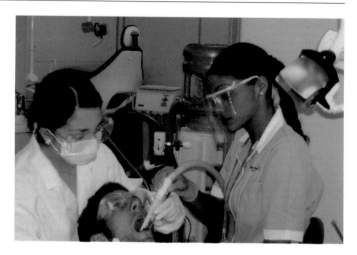

Fig. 2.3 Personal protective equipment/clothing.

PERSONAL PROTECTIVE EQUIPMENT/CLOTHING
To reduce the risk of contamination or injury from debris by inoculation, inhalation, ingestion or absorption through the skin (Figure 2.3).

Clinical uniform/clothing
❏ Clinical uniform/clothing is washed with a suitable detergent at a minimum of 65°C or as recommended by manufacturer.

Gloves
❏ Only worn in the clinical area.
❏ Worn for all clinical procedures.
❏ Discarded after single use.
❏ Changed and discarded if damaged.
❏ Discarded after clinical procedure and new pair donned prior to disinfecting equipment.
❏ Worn when disinfecting equipment and surfaces.
❏ Heavy-duty rubber gloves worn for pre-sterilisation cleaning.

Protective eye wear
- ❏ Only worn in the clinical area.
- ❏ Worn for all clinical procedures by staff and patients.
- ❏ Disinfected after every procedure.
- ❏ Worn for pre-sterilisation cleaning.
- ❏ Worn where there is a risk of debris entering the eye.

Masks/visors
- ❏ Only worn in the clinical area.
- ❏ Worn for all clinical procedures.
- ❏ Worn for pre-sterilisation cleaning.
- ❏ Worn where there is a risk of inhalation/ingestion from substances.
- ❏ Visors may be an alternative to protective eye wear and masks.

Footwear
- ❏ Toe area of shoes should be enclosed.

CLINICAL PROCEDURES
To reduce the risk of transmission during clinical procedures.

- ❏ Have patient medical history ready for review and if necessary revision.
- ❏ Fresh mouth rinse prepared in front of patient.
- ❏ Clean surfaces out of the immediate zone are not touched during procedures.
- ❏ Drawers and cupboards are not ventured into during procedures. If this is necessary, use a hygienic hand rub or remove gloves.
- ❏ Dental syringes are only re-sheathed by dentist/hygienist using appropriate devices.
- ❏ Working areas used during treatment kept to a minimum.

ENVIRONMENT
To ensure the area surrounding the clinical zone is socially clean.

❏ Non-clinical chairs are clean and dust free.
❏ Floors, doors, walls and all areas are checked for cleanliness and cleaned if necessary prior to a session.
❏ Where floors, doors and walls are not to an acceptable standard of cleanliness supervisor/manager is informed.
❏ There are no inappropriate items of equipment in clinical areas.
❏ Surgery is well ventilated by an open window or air-conditioning adjusted as necessary.
❏ Toys are wipeable.

DECONTAMINATION OF EQUIPMENT AND SURFACES
To reduce the number of micro-organisms below the amount able to cause infection through a system of clean and dirty zones.

Start of day
❏ Don gloves, mask, goggles.
❏ Spray, wipe, spray all work surfaces, including dental chair with hard surface disinfectant (or wipes).
❏ Flush through handpiece tubings and 3-in-1 syringe tubes for two to three minutes.
❏ Place disposable sheaths/covers on:
  –spittoon unit;
  –X-ray control unit and cone;
  –computer mouse;
  –handpiece tubings and control unit;
  –3-in-1 syringe tubing;
  –flex for X-ray attachment;
  –light handles;
  –chair headrest.
❏ Prepare ultrasonic fill with detergent.
❏ Daily routine maintenance of autoclave carried out and records completed (see Chapter 1).

Between patients
❏ Remove instruments and place in sink.
❏ Remove all disposable sheaths/covers and mouthwash cup, and place in clinical waste bin.

❏ Spray, wipe, spray all surfaces and equipment (as stated above).
❏ Segregate and dispose of waste.
❏ Replace disposable sheaths/covers.
❏ Replace mouthwash.
❏ Empty and drain ultrasonic bath at end of session where necessary.

End of day
❏ Follow the procedure for 'between patients' above but do not replace disposable sheaths/covers.
❏ Empty and drain ultrasonic bath.
❏ Empty, drain and wipe inside chamber of autoclave.
❏ Clean and rinse water bottle and fill with hypochlorite.
❏ Clean and rinse filters.
❏ Disinfect all tubings.
❏ Clean sinks with hot soapy water and spray with disinfectant.
❏ Place chair in high position.

DECONTAMINATION OF INSTRUMENTS
To ensure there is no risk of transmitting infection from an instrument to a patient.

Pre-sterilisation cleaning
❏ Instruments handled with care, opened/dismantled and placed in ultrasonic basket in sink.
❏ Gently rinse under cold running water to avoid the risk of splashing, and place in bath.
❏ When cycle is complete remove the basket from the tank, place in the sink, rinse the instruments with clean drinking quality water. Heavily soiled instruments may require manual cleaning.
❏ Instruments are removed from basket, inspected for debris if none present, dried prior to autoclaving.
❏ Manual cleaning required where heavy soiling is present or debris remains:

–Hold the part of instrument furthest away from the tip, and scrub gently under running water using a long-handled nylon brush.

–Remember to place brush in autoclave after each use.

Automated cleaning and disinfection removes the need for manual cleaning.

Sterilisation process

❏ Dry instruments, put on autoclave tray across tray ribs, include a Time, Steam and Temperature strip (TST) in every cycle, place in autoclave, commence sterilisation cycle.

❏ Vacuum autoclaves – instruments are packed and wrapped in sterilisation pouches prior to commencing cycle.

❏ Instruments must be used within three hours of sterilisation. For those which are not used within this period, follow the aseptic storage instructions below.

Aseptic storage

Check:

❏ Instruments are dry.

❏ Instrument trays are covered *or* instruments are placed in pouches.

❏ Instrument trays are complete and no item has been removed.

Trays are then placed in storage cupboard.

WASTE DISPOSAL

To ensure waste is disposed of safely and without risk of contamination or injury.

Segregation of waste

Sharps

❏ Sharps box is assembled correctly.

❏ Sharps box stored safely out of patient access.

❏ Sharps box is no more than two-thirds full.

❏ Sharps box is labelled/signed indicating source.

❏ Items marked single use are not used twice (Figure 2.4).

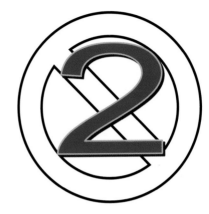

Fig. 2.4 Single-use sign.

Domestic waste
❏ Non-clinical items only are placed in black bags.

Hazardous or clinical waste and non-hazardous waste
❏ Sacks are no more than two-thirds full and tied securely.
❏ Sacks are stored in a designated area inaccessible to unauthorised persons.
❏ Items marked for single use are not used twice.

IMMUNISATION
To ensure dental nurses are appropriately vaccinated against known infectious diseases.

❏ Pre-employment medical screening undertaken and record held in personal file.
❏ Medical screening record includes:
  –Human immunodeficiency virus (HIV)
  –Hepatitis B
  –Hepatitis C
  –Varicella.
❏ Immunisation record relates to the following vaccinations (Figure 2.5):

2

IMMUNISATION RECORD

It is the responsibility of each member of staff to maintain their own personal immunisation record. Each member of staff must provide the employer with accurate and up-to-date information regarding their immune status. The information contained in this record must be kept confidential and only accessible to the employer or other authorised person and the person it relates to, this ensures compliance with the Data Protection Act and Access to Health Records.

NAME:...

VACCINATIONS	SCHEDULE	DATE	EVIDENCE
Rubella (German measles) (OR SEE BELOW)	Administered early teens		
Measles, mumps, rubella (MMR)	Administered during childhood		
Poliomyelitis	Administered during childhood		
Pertussis (whooping cough)	Administered during childhood		

Infection Control **2**

2

Diphtheria	Administered during childhood
Tuberculosis (TB)	Administered during early teens if a negative Heaf's test; BCG scar provides evidence
Tetanus	Administered during childhood immunisation is temporary and may need to be repeated at intervals
Hepatitis B	Recommended for clinical staff, course of injections, followed by blood test. Status checked every five years and booster given if levels fall below 100 IU/ml (Further reading S&M Cross Infection Control) (1) (2) (3) Blood test:

I confirm the above record contains accurate and up-to-date information regarding my immune status.

SIGNATURE:..DATE:.................

Fig. 2.5 Immunisation record.

2

Vaccinations	Route
Rubella or measles, mumps, rubella (MMR)	Intramuscular
MMR	Intramuscular
Poliomyelitis	Oral
Pertussis (whooping cough)	Intramuscular
Diphtheria	Intramuscular
Tuberculosis	Intramuscular
Tetanus	Intramuscular
Hepatitis B	Intramuscular

❏ Results of medical screening confirms protection; *or*
❏ If an individual is not fully protected a risk assessment must be carried out and the outcomes communicated to the individual. Agreement on the actions must be confirmed.

LABORATORY PROCEDURES
To prevent the transmission of infection between internal and external sources.

Despatching items to the laboratory

Alginate impressions
❏ Rinsed and placed in recommended solution for 10 minutes and removed.
❏ Rinsed under running cold water, wrapped and bagged.

Rubber base impressions
❏ Immersed in recommended solution for 10 minutes and bagged.

Appliances/prosthetics
❏ Rinsed under running cold water.
❏ If grossly contaminated place in ultrasonic bath.
❏ Immerse in recommended solution for 10 minutes, rinse and bag.

A statement of disinfection must be attached to all items being sent to the laboratory.

Receiving items from the laboratory

❏ Immerse in recommended solution and rinse prior to placing in patient's mouth.

TRAINING

To ensure dental nurses are aware of and understand the procedures required to prevent the transmission of infection.

Induction

❏ The dental nurse has received information and training on the practice cross-infection control policy (CIC) and procedures.
❏ The dental nurse has received training prior to working in the surgery on the ten key areas of infection control.
❏ The dental nurse's understanding of the ten areas of infection control has been checked and further training provided where appropriate.

Ongoing

❏ The dental nurse's training needs have been reviewed and updated where necessary.

TOP TIPS

1. Adopt universal precautions – the same CIC procedures for all patients and all treatments.
2. Hazardous and non-hazardous waste must not be disposed of in the same sack; seek advice from your waste collection contractors.
3. Carry out routine (frequency determined by policy) infection control self-assessment/audits to ensure standards are being applied and to identify areas for development.
4. Inform your employer if you have any concerns about CIC.
5. Inform your employer if your medical status changes.
6. Obtain the laboratory CIC policy.
7. Familiarise yourself with the practice CIC policy and adhere to it at all times.

LINKS TO OTHER CHAPTERS
- Chapter 1 – Daily Routine Maintenance.
- Chapter 16 – Health and Safety in the Dental Environment.

Initial Examination and Diagnosis

> A thorough examination of the patient's head,
> neck and oral cavity is carried out to assist with
> prevention and early diagnosis of disease.

CLINICAL ASSESSMENT OF A PATIENT'S ORAL AND
GENERAL HEALTH

The dental team have an interest in the oral health and general
well-being of their patients. An assessment of the intra-oral structures, extra-oral features and general health of the patient is
carried out routinely.

Purpose of clinical assessment
❏ To confirm that the patient is dentally fit.
❏ To determine and agree the necessary treatment.
❏ To detect early changes in a patient's condition.
❏ To carry out further investigations.
❏ To reduce the risk of conditions becoming more serious.
❏ To identify anything that could contraindicate dental
treatment.
❏ To help prevent dental disease.

Routine examination and assessment
Although the frequency of a patient's attendance will depend
upon several factors each time a patient attends for their routine
examination the following assessment should be undertaken:

❏ the patient's personal details;
❏ a full medical history (Figure 3.1);
❏ review their dental history and identify any new problems;
❏ examine the status:

MEDICAL HEALTH HISTORY QUESTIONNAIRE

TO THE PATIENT: Please complete this questionnaire as honestly and accurately as possible. The clinician will discuss your responses prior to any treatment being administered. The information contained within this document is confidential in order to comply with the Data Protection Act 1998.

NAME: **DATE OF BIRTH:**   **NI NUMBER:**

GP/DOCTOR:

(1) Have you had any operations since your last visit?

(2) Have you had an illness or injury since your last visit?

(3) Have you attended a doctor, hospital, clinic or specialist since your last visit?

(4) Are you taking any medication?

MEDICAL CONDITIONS: Do you have or have you had any problems with the following?:

(5) Chest, e.g. asthma or bronchitis:

(6) Heart, e.g. angina, rheumatic fever or replacement valve:

(7) Blood pressure: _____

(8) Circulation, e.g. anaemia or haemophilia: _____

(9) Diabetes: _____

(10) Digestion, e.g. ulcers, jaundice or colitis: _____

(11) Kidneys: _____

(12) Epilepsy: _____

(13) Arthritis: _____

(14) Skin, e.g. ulcers or eczema: _____

(15) Allergies, e.g. penicillin, rubber products, metals or food: _____

HEALTH CONDITIONS

(16) Could you be pregnant? _____

(17) Have you ever had problems with anaesthetic, e.g. inhalation, local or general? _____

(18) Do you have any history of family illnesses? _____

(19) Have you been exposed to any infections, e.g. HIV, TB or hepatitis? _____

Fig. 3.1 *Continued overleaf*

SMOKING AND DRINKING HABITS

(20) Have you smoked any form of tobacco within the past three years?

(21) If you previously smoked and given up when did you give up?:

(22) Do you currently use any form of tobacco? If yes what form and how much?

(22) How many years have you been using tobacco for?

(23) Do you chew betel nut or any other substance?

(24) If you drink alcohol how much do you drink per week?

(25) What type of alcohol do you drink?

OTHER HABITS

(26) Do you snore when sleeping?

(27) Do you grind or clench your teeth?

(27) Do you chew the inside of your cheeks or lips?

ANY FURTHER DETAILS – please add anything else you feel is relevant to your medical health, e.g. if you have experienced any problems when undergoing dental or medical treatment:

_____

_____

_____

_____

CLINICIAN'S COMMENTS – NAME OF CLINICIAN _____

_____

_____

_____

_____

Signed by Patient:_____ Date_____

Signed by Clinician_____ Date_____

Fig. 3.1 Medical history form.

–of existing teeth and restorations;
–occlusion;
–appliances.

Status of intra-oral soft tissues
This includes:

–tongue;
–floor of mouth;
–uvula;
–palate;
–oral mucosa;
–periodontal structures;
–any indication of halitosis.

Ask the patient if they have any problems, i.e. sore throat, pain, difficulty with swallowing, etc. Special solutions/mouth rinses may be used which will stain any suspicious areas.

Status of extra-oral features
This includes:

–lips;
–skin colour;
–blemishes, moles, lesions;
–lymph nodes;
–face shape;
–any swelling.

A visual examination of the head, neck and facial area should be carried out, and careful palpation with the hands and finger tips of the lymph nodes in the neck.

A detailed and thorough assessment is vital for the detection of any suspicious lesions that could be early signs of oral cancer. If the dentist detects an abnormality referral for diagnosis and treatment is essential (Figure 3.2).

'At-risk' groups for oral cancer are:

❑ over 40 years of age;
❑ smokers;

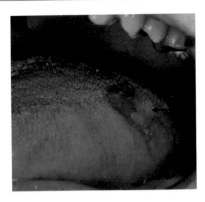

Fig. 3.2 Early signs of oral cancer. Arrow shows cancerous lesion on tongue.

❏ regular heavy drinkers of alcohol especially those who smoke as well;
❏ those who chew tobacco or betel nut;
❏ previous history of cancer;
❏ immunocompromised state.

The dental nurse's role in initial examination and assessment

❏ Universal cross-infection control procedures must be adopted throughout all examinations/assessments.
❏ Make available all records relating to the patient including:
  – previous medical and dental histories;
  – new medical history form;
  – radiographs;
  – photographs;
  – study models;
  – referral letters;
  – general practitioner or occupational health letters/reports;
  – hygienist letters/reports.
❏ Lay out the required equipment and instruments as follows (Figure 3.3):
  – mouth mirror;
  – right-angled probe;
  – college tweezers;

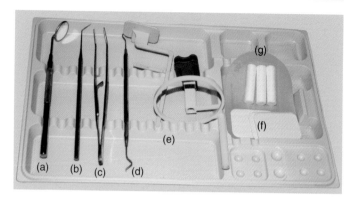

Fig. 3.3 Initial examination/assessment tray. (a) Mouth mirror; (b) right-angled probe; (c) college tweezers; (d) Briault probe; (e) X-ray holders; (f) X-ray films; (g) cotton wool rolls.

  –Briault probe;
  –X-ray films and holder (taking X-rays must be justified);
  –Cotton wool rolls (moisture control).

All of the above are placed on the examination tray. Additional items may also be required, e.g.:

  –aspirator tip;
  –mouth rinse and tissue;
  –alginate impression material, impression trays, mixing bowl and spatula (if study models required);
  –articulating paper;
  –sheet wax;
  –pulp testing – ethyl chloride, gutta percha or electric pulp tester.

Communication with the patient
• Explain the procedure to the patient (avoid using jargon), provide support and reassurance as required by each patient.

- Assist the patient with the completion of medical history form if necessary.
- Provide protective spectacles and bib for patient.
- Provide gloves, mask and protective spectacles for dentist and dental nurse.
- Anticipate clinician's needs and pass instruments and equipment as required.
- **Take valid, accurate, reliable, current and sufficient notes and present to dentist for verification.**
- Use a standard chart to record the initial examination and assessment.

The system most commonly used in the UK is one where teeth are numbered 1 to 8 in adult dentition and A to E in primary dentition (Figure 3.4). There is also a two-digit system, the Federation Dentaire Internationale (FDI; International Dental Federation) system (Figure 3.5).

PERIODONTAL EXAMINATION AND ASSESSMENT
This is carried out by either the dentist or the hygienist.

The dental nurse's role in periodontal examination and assessment

❏ Make available all records relating to the patient as detailed in the initial examination and assessment.
❏ Lay out the required instruments as follows (Figure 3.6):

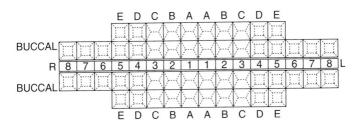

Fig. 3.4 Standard UK charting.

FDI — International Dental Federation

International system of charting used mostly outside Great Britain.

Simplifies dental data in computer programs.

FDI Two-digit system

PERMANENT TEETH — Quadrants are numbered: 1–4.

Charting in a clockwise DIRECTION.

Quadrant 1	Quadrant 2
Quadrant 4	Quadrant 3

Quadrants number first, then followed by tooth number.

18 17 16 15 14 13 12 11	21 22 23 24 25 26 27 28
48 47 46 45 44 43 42 41	31 32 33 34 35 36 37 38

PRIMARY TEETH – Quadrants are numbered: 5–8.

Quadrant 5	Quadrant 6
Quadrant 8	Quadrant 7

Quadrants number first, then followed by tooth number.

55 54 53 52 51	61 62 63 64 65
85 84 83 82 81	71 72 73 74 75

Number pronounced separately, e.g.: Five–Five *not* Fifty-five

Fig. 3.5 FDI charting.

–mouth mirror;
–Basic Periodontal Examination (BPE) probe;
–Williams periodontal pocket measuring probe;
–calculus probe;
–disclosing solution/tablets;
–X-ray films and holder (taking X-rays must be justified);
–cotton wool rolls (moisture control).

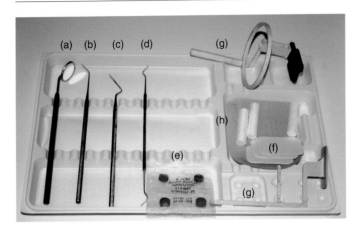

Fig. 3.6 Periodontal examination/assessment tray. (a) Mouth mirror; (b) BPE probe; (c) Williams probe; (d) calculus probe; (e) disclosing tablets; (f) X-ray films; (g) X-ray film holders; (h) cotton wool rolls.

All of the above are placed on the periodontal examination tray, additional items may also be required, e.g.:

   –aspirator tip;
   –mouth wash and tissue.
❏ Provide demonstration models, diagrams, charts or pictures to communicate findings to patient.
❏ Charting of plaque and bleeding scores and pocket depth.
❏ A BPE chart can be used (Figure 3.7).
❏ Follow the actions detailed in the section 'Communication with the patient'.

ORTHODONTIC EXAMINATION AND ASSESSMENT

At the initial appointment the cause of the malocclusion will be established and a detailed assessment carried out. Malocclusion is classified as follows: Class I, Class II division 1, Class II division 2, Class III (Figure 3.8).

The clinician/dentist may also use the Dental Health Component of the Index of Orthodontic Treatment Need (IOTN) to

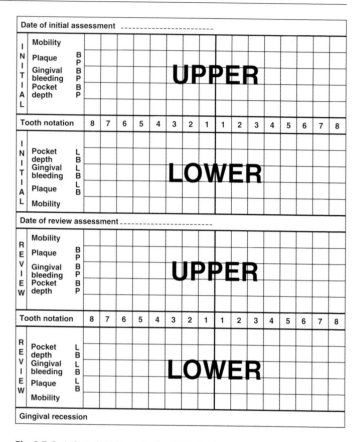

Fig. 3.7 Basic Periodontal Examination (BPE) charting.

assess the level of malocclusion. The following grading system is used:

Grade 5 – Extreme/need treatment (see examples below)

- Impeded eruption of teeth (except third molars) due to crowding, displacement, the presence of supernumerary teeth, retained deciduous teeth and any pathological cause.
- Increased overjet greater than 9 mm.

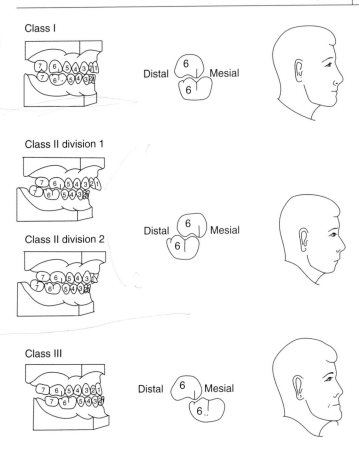

Fig. 3.8 Classification of malocclusion.

Grade 4 – Severe/need treatment (see examples below)

- Less extensive developmental absence of teeth.
- Increased overjet greater than 6 mm but less than or equal to 9 mm.

Grade 3 – Moderate/borderline need (see examples below)

- Increased overjet greater than 3.5 mm but less than or equal to 6 mm with incompetent lips.
- Lateral or anterior open bite greater than 2 mm but less than or equal to 4 mm.

Grade 2 – Mid/little need (see examples below)

- Increased overjet greater than 3.5 mm but less than or equal to 6 mm with competent lips.
- Increased overbite greater than or equal to 3.5 mm with gingival contact.

Grade 1 – No need (see example below)

- Extremely minor malocclusions including contact point displacements less than 1 mm.

Causes of malocclusion
These fall into two categories – general and local factors.

General factors
These affect the development of the dental arches as a whole:

- hereditary factors;
- structure of facial skeleton;
- shape and activity of facial soft tissues;
- size and shape of teeth;
- abnormality, e.g. cleft palate;
- injury at birth;
- disease or injury.

Local factors
These affect the development of the dental arches at specific points:

- bottle feeding;
- missing teeth;
- supernumerary teeth;
- premature loss or prolonged retention of deciduous teeth;

- impaction of teeth;
- loss of permanent teeth;
- lip and tongue behaviour;
- thumb sucking;
- localised disease, e.g. tumour or injury.

Both parent and patient (if patient is under 16 years) must be involved at the initial assessment stage in order to gain co-operation and agreement.

Detailed orthodontic examination

Extra-oral
Skeletal jaw relationship, and shape, form and activity of lips.

Intra-oral
General examination of all teeth, and shape, form and activity of tongue and swallowing action, tooth contact on opening and closing, measurement of overbite, overjet, tooth width and spaces between teeth.

If the patient is ready for treatment the following procedures are undertaken:

- X-rays to distinguish the presence and position of unerupted teeth, supernumeraries and any abnormalities.
- Photographs (extra-oral and intra-oral views).
- Study models and wax bite to show teeth in occlusion and to assist with treatment planning.

The dental nurse's role in orthodontic assessment
❏ Make available all records relating to the patient detailed in the initial examination and assessment.
❏ Lay out the following instruments/equipment:
   –mirror;
   –right-angled probe;
   –BPE probe;
   –college tweezers;
   –dividers;
   –calliper gauge;

−X-ray films and holder (taking X-rays must be justified);
−cotton wool rolls (moisture control).

All of the above are placed on the orthodontic examination tray. The following additional items may also be required:

−camera;
−alginate impression material, impression trays, mixing bowl, spatula and laboratory ticket;
−sheet wax;
−aspirator tip;
−mouth rinse and tissue;

❑ prepare X-ray films and patient;
❑ take photographs if competent to do so;
❑ reassure and support patient throughout;
❑ chart the periodontal status on dictation from the clinician;
❑ chart present, missing and genetically absent teeth on dictation from the clinician;
❑ present the records to the clinician for verification;
❑ follow the actions detailed in the section 'Communication with the patient'.

TOP TIPS

1. The dental nurse must ensure dental records are valid, accurate, reliable, current and sufficient and presented to the clinician/dentist or hygienist for verification.
2. Recording of all information is of paramount importance, as it could be used in a clinician's defence in a case of litigation.
3. Consent to treatment from the patient, or parent if the patient is under 16 years, must be obtained and the relevant forms signed prior to any treatment being undertaken.

LINKS TO OTHER CHAPTERS
- Chapter 4 – Dental Radiography.
- Chapter 12 – Dental Implants.
- Chapter 14 – Managing Dental Records.

Dental Radiography

4

Dental nurses play a vital role in contributing to
the quality assurance of dental radiographs.

ESSENTIAL LEGAL REQUIREMENTS

It is of utmost importance that dental nurses are aware of and
comply with the rules and regulations relating to dental radiography to protect themselves, their colleagues and patients. Two
specific regulations relate to the use of X-ray equipment in dental
practices: the Ionising Radiations Regulations 1999 and the Ionising Radiation (Medical Exposure) Regulations 2000.

Ionising Radiations Regulations 1999 (IRR 99)

These Regulations came into force on 1 January 2000, replacing
the Ionising Radiations Regulations 1985. The IRR 99 primarily
deals with the **protection of employees** from ionising radiation
in the work place and the **protection of patients from the X-ray
equipment**. Under the Regulations dentists are classed as radiation employers and are required to comply with the following:

❏ **Notification** to the Health and Safety Executive (HSE), using
a form F9 or equivalent, of the installation and use of X-ray
equipment. If certain changes occur, HSE is notified, e.g.
change of ownership.
❏ **Prior (pro-active) risk assessment** when new X-ray equipment is planned, existing equipment is modified and when
equipment is re-located.

❑ Have systems in place to **restrict exposure** through adhering to annual Dose Limitations.

❑ **Maintenance** of X-ray equipment through critical examinations and acceptance testing.

❑ **Contingency plans** must be in place to address foreseeable accidents arising from the use of X-ray equipment.

❑ **A radiation protection advisor** (RPA) must be appointed in writing, to provide advice and act as a consultant. The RPA will be appointed externally and all advice given must be obtained in writing.

❑ **Information, instruction and training** must be provided to all staff directly involved in the taking and processing of radiographs and those not directly associated with the activities.

❑ **Designation** of 'controlled areas' around the X-ray equipment.

❑ **Display written Local Rules** to ensure that exposure to staff is restricted.

❑ **One or more radiation protection supervisors** (RPSs) must be appointed to assist with compliance. An RPS can be a dentist or dental nurse, the appointee must be competent to supervise the arrangements set out in local rules.

❑ Designate staff as '**classified persons**' if they are required to enter the controlled area, however, this is unlikely to be required.

❑ A **Quality Assurance Programme** must be in place to ensure all radiographs are to the required standard and radiation doses are controlled.

IRR 99 also places legal requirements on employees as follows:

❑ **The duties of employees** are to ensure that:
   –they do not expose themselves or others to unnecessary doses;
   –they exercise care and attention at all times;
   –they report to their employer if they suspect any over-exposure;
   –they report to their employer any accident involving the X-ray equipment.

Ionising Radiation (Medical Exposure) Regulations 2000 IR (ME) R2000

These Regulations came into force on 13 May 2000 replacing the Ionising (Protection of Persons Undergoing Medical Examination or Treatment) Regulations 1988 (POPUMET). The IR (ME) R2000 primarily deals with the **restriction of doses to patients from medical exposure**. Under the Regulations employing dentists are required to comply with the following:

- ❏ Provide **written procedures** for the taking of dental X-rays to ensure patient safety.
- ❏ **Define the duties** performed by the key people appointed by the employer who are involved in the medical exposure.
- ❏ Provide **justification** as to why the medical exposure is required.
- ❏ Ensure all doses are kept as low as reasonably practicable to ensure protection of all through '**optimisation**' of exposure.
- ❏ Carry out **clinical audits** to ensure the ionising radiation programme is being effectively implemented.
- ❏ Identify the need for and involvement of a **medical physics expert (MPE)** to advise on patient doses.
- ❏ Keep an up-to-date **equipment inventory** of each item of X-ray equipment.
- ❏ Ensure that IRMER practitioners and operators receive adequate and appropriate **training**.

Dental nurses have a legal responsibility to ensure they comply with employee duties and co-operate with the employer to assist them in meeting their legal duties.

TYPES OF RADIOGRAPHS AND THE REASONS FOR USE

Two types of radiograph are used in dental surgeries, these are known as 'intra-oral' and 'extra-oral':

Intra-oral radiographs

Intra-oral radiographs are positioned inside the mouth to show an image of a single tooth or a few teeth over a small area. This type of X-ray consists of the following (Figure 4.1):

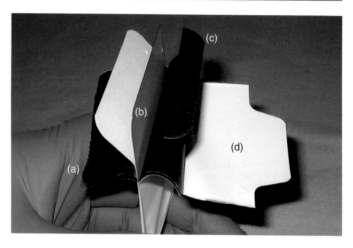

Fig. 4.1 X-ray film packet. (a) Lead foil; (b) X-ray film; (c) black paper; (d) plastic outer wrapping.

- Plastic outer wrapping – white in colour and waterproof (wraps around the entire contents)
- Black paper – prevents light filtering through
- X-ray film – light green colour
- Lead foil – absorbs radiation and prevents scatter.

Types and reasons for use
Please note the most common uses are listed, however, this may differ in practice.

Periapical – shows anatomy of whole tooth including, apex, pulp, crown, supporting bone. Provides a detailed view of a small area (Figure 4.2). **Reason for use** – root canal treatment, periodontal assessment, apical condition and recurrent caries.

Bitewing – shows the crowns of upper and lower teeth (Figure 4.3). **Reason for use** – vertical bitewing shows periodontal disease and bone loss in posterior teeth, horizontal bitewing shows inter-

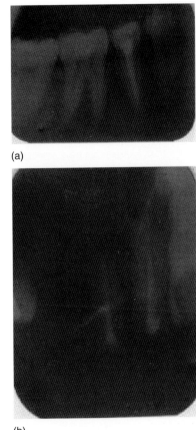

(a)

4

Fig. 4.2 (a,b) Periapical
radiographs.   (b)

proximal caries, early caries, caries under existing restoration,
edges of restorations and bone levels.

Occlusal – larger than periapical and bitewing, shows upper or
lower view of bone and teeth in maxilla or mandible (Figure 4.4).
Reasons for use – unerupted teeth, supernumerary teeth and
cysts.

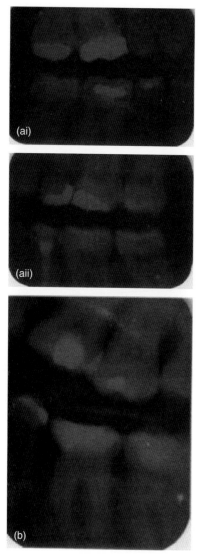

Fig. 4.3 (a) Horizontal bitewing radiographs. (b) Vertical bitewing radiograph.

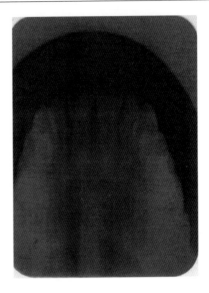

Fig. 4.4 Occlusal radiograph.

The dental nurse's role in intra-oral radiographs

❑ Comply with the Quality Assurance Programme.
❑ Assist clinician by carrying out the following:

  –Lay out X-ray films appropriate to procedure.
  –Ask patient to remove personal items – removable dental prosthesis and tongue jewellery, place in secure receptacle and confirm contents with patient.
  –Seat patient in upright position and provide instruction on remaining still during exposure.
  –Place film and holder in patient's mouth (**only** if competent to do so) (Figure 4.5).
  –Position X-ray tube head correctly, depending on techniques being used, **only** if competent to do so.
  –Activate warning light to inform exposure to radiation is taking place or prevent entry to controlled area.
  –Connect X-ray set to electricity supply.
  –Following exposure deactivate warning light or re-enter controlled area.

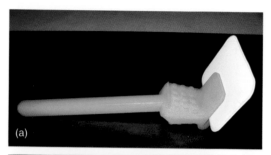

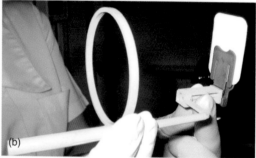

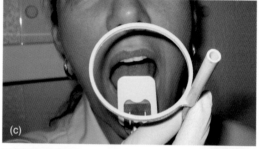

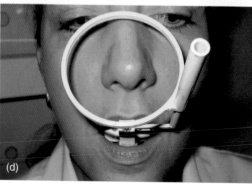

–Remove film and holder, disinfect and dry prior to processing.

–Return personal items to patient and confirm all items are returned.

–Process radiograph (see processing).

–Make valid, accurate, reliable, current and sufficient notes and present to clinician for verification.

Extra-oral radiographs

Types and reasons for use
Please note the most common uses are listed, however, this may differ in practice.

Orthopantomograph (OPG) – shows a panoramic view of both upper and lower jaws and all teeth both erupted and unerupted. The film is contained inside a **cassette** where it is sandwiched between two white intensifying screens which reduce the radiation dose and give off light on exposure to radiation, this enhances and produces the image (Figure 4.6). **Reasons for use** – assess overall development of dentition, bone levels for periodontal assessment, detect retained roots, cysts, abnormalities, alignment of temporomandibular joints, position of inferior dental canal and maxillary antrum.

Lateral oblique – shows a right or left side view of the posterior region and part of the jaw. Once again a cassette is used to house the film, the patient holds the cassette against the side of the face where it rests on the ramus of mandible and cheek (Figure 4.7). **Reasons for use** – determine position of unerupted third molars, has limited use in dentistry today as OPG (see above) is more frequently used.

Fig. 4.5 Placing film and holder in the patient's mouth. (a) Film and bitewing holder; (b) film and periapical holder; (c) placing film and holder in mouth; (d) film and holder in place ready to take X-ray.

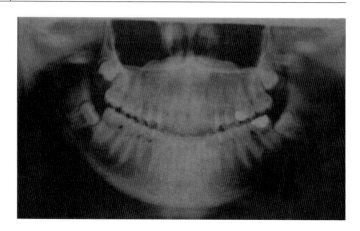

Fig. 4.6 Orthopantomograph.

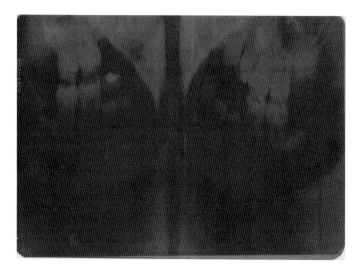

Fig. 4.7 Lateral oblique radiograph.

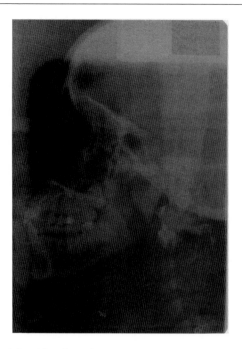

Fig. 4.8 Cephalometric radiograph.

Cephalometric – shows views of the whole skull, most commonly used by orthodontists and oral surgeons. A cephalostat machine is used which takes side and front views. Tracings are done to measure and analyse bone and soft tissues to help with diagnosis and treatment planning. Tracings are then compared at stages (Figure 4.8). **Reasons for use** – determine the severity and degree of malocclusion and position of facial alignment.

The dental nurse's role in extra-oral radiographs
❏ Comply with the Quality Assurance Programme.
❏ Assist clinician by carrying out the following:
   –Lay out X-ray films required for procedure and place in appropriate cassette.

- Ask patient to remove all personal items – removable dental prosthesis, tongue jewellery, ear and nose rings and necklaces, place in secure receptacle and confirm contents with patient.
- Seat or stand patient in appropriate position and provide instruction on remaining still during exposure.
- OPG and cephalometric – place cassette in X-ray machine (**only** if competent to do so).
- Lateral oblique – position cassette and X-ray tube head correctly (**only** if competent to do so).
- Activate warning light to inform exposure to radiation is taking place or prevent entry to controlled area.
- Connect X-ray set to electricity supply.
- Following exposure deactivate warning light and re-enter controlled area.
- Return personal items to patient and confirm all items are returned.
- Process radiograph (see processing).
- Make valid, accurate, reliable, current and sufficient notes and present to clinician for verification.

PROCESSING DENTAL RADIOGRAPHS

A key principle of the **Quality Assurance Programme** is to ensure radiographs are of good diagnostic quality, it is important that processing is carried out correctly in order to avoid unnecessary retakes.

Manual processing and darkroom procedures

This method of processing is used less frequently today as more practices now use an automatic processer. However, it is important the following rules are applied with all manual processing:

❏ Darkrooms must be free from outside light and well ventilated.
❏ X-ray films should only be exposed to a safelight for short periods.

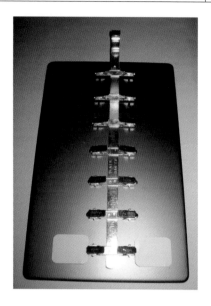

Fig. 4.9 X-ray film hanger.

❏ Safelights should be at a suitable distance from the working area and correct filters installed.

❏ Warning light should be displayed outside the room to prevent people entering.

❏ Arrange darkroom into two zones – wet and dry processing.

❏ Surfaces must be kept dry and clean to prevent contamination from spilt solutions.

❏ Check film speed to determine correct processing times.

❏ Clip X-ray film packet to hanger and record orientation (do this outside the room) (Figure 4.9).

❏ Check levels of developer, fixer and water and replenish or change if required.

❏ Check temperature of solutions (according to manufacturer's instructions) and use immersion heater if necessary.

❏ Once inside the room ensure hands are dry to prevent moisture contamination.

❏ Unclip films in turn from hanger and remove contents from packet, discard outer wrapping, black paper, lead foil and re-clip film to hanger, if using extra-oral cassette remove film from cassette.

❏ Hold films at the edge between thumb and forefinger to prevent prints on radiograph.

❏ Set timer according to manufacturer's instructions for the first **four** stages:

–**Develop** – immerse films in developing solutions for speci-fied time, move film around for even coverage and to prevent air bubbles, then cover with lid.

–**Wash** – rinse films in water for approximately 15 seconds, this stops the developing action.

–**Fix** – place washed films in fixing tank for specified time, this will complete the fixation.

–**Wash** – rinse radiographs thoroughly to remove all chemicals.

–**Dry** – hang films to dry in a dust-free area, ensuring they don't overlap or touch one another.

❏ Switch on overhead light, switch off safe light.

❏ Remove all debris and ensure room is left clean and free from contamination.

Automatic processing

This is carried out using a self-contained sealed unit consisting of developer, water and fixing tanks. The films are dried inside the machine. The unit must be maintained frequently, the rollers washed and cleaned, chemical and water levels checked, replen-ished and changed regularly.

Other forms of processing

Digital processing

The two methods of processing already mentioned rely on films and processing solutions. This method uses a computer to capture the image, which is instantly stored in the memory and displayed on the monitor. The image is immediately available.

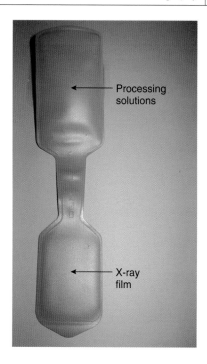

Fig. 4.10 Instant X-ray film.

Instant processing (Figure 4.10)

This method is no longer widely used due to practices now having automatic or digital processing facilities. However, in instances where such processors are not available or where equipment is not working instant processing is a useful alternative. The film and processing solutions are contained within a plastic outer wrapping, the film is at one end and the solution at the other, when the X-ray has been taken the solution is 'squeezed' down into the film compartment to develop the radiograph. The plastic outer wrapping is then removed to expose the processed radiograph.

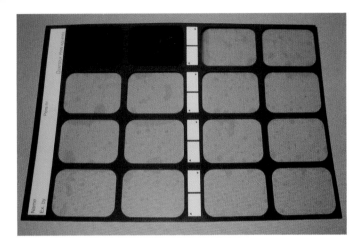

Fig. 4.11 Mounting radiographs.

CARE OF EQUIPMENT

Care of X-ray films
❏ Store in cool, dry area away from X-ray equipment.
❏ Do not store OPG boxes on top of one another to avoid the risk of squashing the emulsion on the film or the emulsified layer.
❏ Carry out strict stock control, use oldest films first, and do not use after expiry date.

Care of radiographs

Mounting (Figure 4.11)
❏ Pimple towards you, bump side up.
❏ Ascertain left or right side.
❏ Place in orientated positions.
❏ Mount must be labelled and dated.

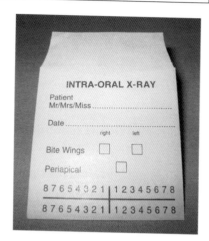

INTRA-ORAL X-RAY

Patient
Mr/Mrs/Miss ....

Date ....

	right	left
Bite Wings	☐	☐
Periapical	☐	

8 7 6 5 4 3 2 1 | 1 2 3 4 5 6 7 8
8 7 6 5 4 3 2 1 | 1 2 3 4 5 6 7 8

Fig. 4.12 Storing radiographs.

Storing (Figure 4.12)
❏ Ensure patient's name, reference, date taken, tooth/teeth X-rayed are clearly recorded.
❏ Radiographs must be stored securely to comply with data protection and avoid losses.

Care of extra-oral cassettes
❏ Never leave cassettes open when not in use, dust may settle and intensifying screens may be contaminated.
❏ Clean intensifying screen regularly with solution recommended by manufacturer.
❏ Never scratch intensifying screens to remove any dirt.
❏ Store cassettes to avoid the risk of damage, i.e. place on stable surfaces.

Care of chemical processing solutions
❏ Prepare to manufacturer's instructions.
❏ Use at the correct temperature.
❏ Use test objects/strips to monitor for deterioration, i.e. strip too light, chemicals need changing.

❏ Change or replenish frequently according to results of tests and or usage.

❏ Store away from heat, in an upright position, at floor level.

❏ Dispose of waste chemicals through a collection agency – do not pour into main drainage.

Care of X-ray equipment

❏ Keep an equipment log of all equipment and maintenance.

❏ Carry out routine checks to ensure equipment is functioning correctly and safely to include:

–warning lights and audible alarms;

–safety devices;

–performance of the counterbalance of the tube head.

❏ Ensure equipment is clean to reduce contamination.

FAULTY IMAGES

Fault	Cause	Prevention
Bright image (Figure 4.13)	Under-exposed Out of date developer	Adjust exposure time Change developer
Dark image (Figure 4.14)	Over-exposed Over-developed	Adjust exposure time Reduce time and or temperature
Partly blank (Figure 4.15)	Incorrect angulation	Direct beam to middle of film
Blurred image (Figure 4.16)	Patient or machine moved	Ensure patient is fully informed Use fast film to reduce exposure time Ensure routine machine maintenance
Bright spots (Figure 4.17)	Fixer splash on film	Keep darkroom areas clean and dry
	Inadequate washing	Wash thoroughly after fixing

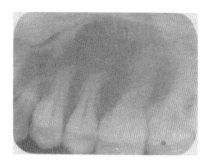

Fig. 4.13 A bright image.

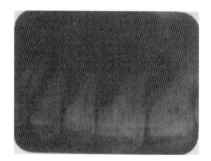

Fig. 4.14 A dark image.

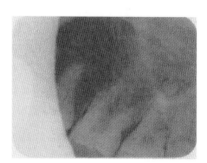

Fig. 4.15 Partly blank image.

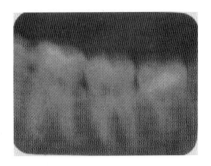

Fig. 4.16 Blurred image.

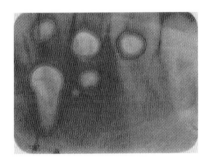

Fig. 4.17 Bright spots on image.

	Grease/oil on hands	Wash and dry hands before processing
Black lines (Figure 4.18)	Finger nail marks	Handle film gently
	Bending in patient's mouth	Ensure patient is not biting unnecessarily
Dark patch (Figure 4.19)	Film in contact with another	Agitate films in fixing bath
Bright patches (Figure 4.20)	Temperature of solutions too high	Check temperature and reduce

QUALITY ASSURANCE AND CONTROL

The overall aim of the Quality Assurance Programme is to ensure that diagnostic images are produced to a consistently high quality

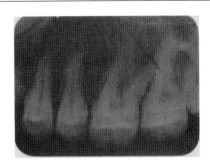

Fig. 4.18 Black line on image.

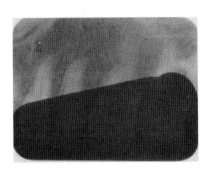

Fig. 4.19 Dark patch on image.

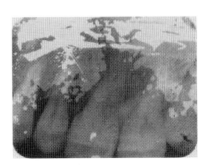

Fig. 4.20 Extensive bright patches on image.

which provide adequate information at the lowest possible cost with the least exposure of radiation to the patient. Dental nurses must both understand and follow the procedures contained in the dental radiology Quality Assurance Programme. The procedures should be in writing and made available to all members of staff. Listed below are the six areas contained in the Quality Assurance Programme:

Staff training and continuing education

A register should be kept of all staff involved with any aspect of radiology including those who take X-rays and process films. Record the following:

- individual's specific responsibilities;
- the dates and type/nature of training received;
- training review dates (every five years).

Dental nurses have a responsibility to ensure they record all relevant details and attend training reviews.

Image quality and film reject analysis

❏ Image quality must be monitored on a regular basis.
❏ Compare quality of every radiograph to a high standard reference film.
❏ Investigate any deterioration in quality and determine corrective action.
❏ Use minimum targets to assess the quality of radiographic images.
❏ Record outcomes and action taken of the above.
❏ Collect and analyse all rejected radiographs, determine the cause and instigate corrective action.

Working procedures

❏ Ensure you have access to and understand the 'Radiation Protection File'.
❏ Follow the written working procedures for care of equipment, X-ray films, radiographs, chemicals, etc. as listed previously.
❏ Take part in reviewing all procedures at least every 12 months with your employer.

X-ray equipment
❏ Carry out routine equipment checks as described in Care of X-ray equipment, and record details.

Darkroom, X-ray films and processing
❏ Carry out regular checks on the darkroom to ensure it is fit for the purpose (see Manual processing and darkroom procedures).
❏ Ensure films are stored, handled and controlled (see Care of X-ray films).
❏ Follow procedures for care of cassettes, as previously described.
❏ Ensure correct processing of films and care of processing equipment as previously described.

4

Audit
❏ A review of all areas within the Quality Assurance Programme to ensure that they are compliant with the required standards is required annually.
❏ Audits should be carried out by the person with overall control for the Quality Assurance Programme.
❏ The audit should be undertaken by an independent auditor every three years.

DENTAL NURSES AS OPERATORS
Dental nurses may act as **operators**, therefore, undertaking **all or part** of the practical aspect of dental radiography. Practical aspects include:

❏ patient identification;
❏ positioning the film, the patient and X-ray tube head;
❏ setting the exposure;
❏ pressing the exposure button to expose the radiograph;
❏ processing the films;
❏ clinically evaluating the radiographs;
❏ exposing the test object.

If you carry out all or some of the above procedures you must be adequately trained to undertake that specific role, and take part in continuing education every five years. Training must be recorded.

ADVICE AND INFORMATION

The National Radiological Protection Board (NRPB) merged with the Health Protection Agency (HPA) on 1 April 2005 and resulted in a new division being formed to address radiation protection. The Radiation Protection Division of the HPA provides a range of services including:

- research concentrating on the risks of radiation;
- identification of necessary protection;
- delivery of training;
- acts in an advisory role;
- provides the services of an RPA and an MPE.

TOP TIPS

1. Adopt a practical approach to ionising radiation protection by following the six areas of the Quality Assurance Programme.
2. Talk to your employer if you are in doubt about any aspect of ionising radiation and report any concerns.
3. Use FIFO for controlling stocks of X-ray films and chemicals (First In First Out).
4. Ensure you are appropriately trained to carry out any practical aspect of dental radiography.

LINKS TO OTHER CHAPTERS
- Chapter 3 – Initial Diagnosis.
- Chapter 16 – Health and Safety in the Dental Environment.

Root Canal Treatment

5

STAGE 1

Root canal treatment is usually carried out over two visits.

The aim of the first stage is to remove infection and clean and shape the canal ready for filling at the second stage (Figure 5.1).

The procedure

(1) Having identified the need for root canal treatment the dentist will need to gain access to the canal, this involves drilling through the occlusal surface of the tooth and will require the dental nurse to aspirate.

(2) The dead nerve tissue is extirpated (removed) using a barbed broach. A fine root canal file is inserted into the canal and an X-ray taken to determine the canal length.

(3) The canal is then cleaned and shaped using root canal files of increasing size and decreasing length until the root canal file is used at a length 3mm shorter than the working length (this is called the step-back technique – see below).

(4) Once the canal is shaped and cleaned it will need to be washed and dried using a hypodermic syringe filled with saline and paper points until the dentist is satisfied that the infection has been removed.

(5) The canal is then dressed with an antiseptic/anti-bacterial agent and a temporary filling material placed in the access cavity.

(6) The patient is given a second appointment for the canals to be filled and treatment completed.

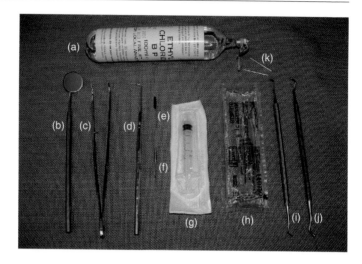

Fig. 5.1 Instruments and materials required for stage 1. (a) Ethyl chloride; (b) mirror; (c) tweezers; (d) probe; (e) barbed broach; (f) Gates Glidden bur; (g) hypodermic syringe; (h) saline; (i) flat plastic; (j) plugger; (k) paper points. Additional equipment: hypodermic needle, sedative dressing material, cotton wool pledgets, periapical film.

Step-back technique

Once the apex has been located, the canal is flared by increasing file size and decreasing length by 1 mm. For example, a 22-mm canal would be flared using a size 15 file at 22 mm, followed by a size 20 file at 21 mm, a size 25 file at 20 mm and a size 30 file at 19 mm. After a 3 mm decrease, the canal is flared enough.

STAGE 2

The aim of the second stage is to ensure the canal is infection free and to fill the canal and access cavity (Figure 5.2).

The procedure

(1) The dressings placed at the first visit are removed and the canal is washed and dried.

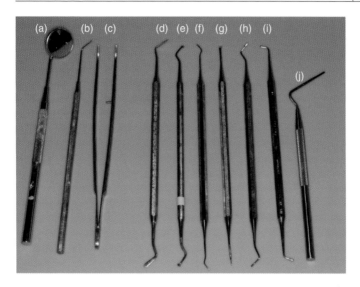

Fig. 5.2 Instruments and materials required for stage 2. (a) Mirror; (b) probe; (c) tweezers; (d) carver; (e) excavator; (f) excavator; (g) flat plastic; (h) plugger; (i) pear-shaped plugger; (j) lateral condenser. Additional equipment: hypodermic syringe and needle, saline, paper points, endodontic files, gutta percha points, root canal sealant, periapical film, filling material.

(2) If all infection has been eliminated the canal can be filled using gutta percha (GP) points and a zinc oxide and eugenol dressing material.

(3) A master GP point is placed in the canal at the initial length used at the beginning of the step-back technique. (Using the example in stage 1 this would be a size 15 point at 22 mm.) An X-ray is taken to ensure that the GP point has reached the end of the canal.

(4) If this is all satisfactory, then accessory GP points are dipped in the zinc oxide and eugenol dressing and packed into the canal using a lateral condenser until the dentist is happy that the canal is free from air pockets.

(5) The protruding ends of the GP points are then removed using a heated instrument and the access cavity filled using a permanent filling material and a final X-ray taken.

OTHER ENDODONTIC TREATMENTS
• Pulpotomy – this is usually performed on children and involves removing only the part of the pulp that is in the pulp chamber.
• Pulpectomy – the removal of pulp tissue. Also referred to as extirpation and usually followed by full root canal treatment.
• Apicectomy – a surgical procedure where infection is removed from the apical end of the root canal (see Chapter 7, Minor Oral Surgery).

TOP TIPS
1. Refer to the records made at the first visit to identify the correct master GP point to be used.
2. Keep a record of the files used and at what length in the patient's notes as this will help at subsequent visits.

Extractions

6

Teeth are extracted for many reasons, e.g. if they are grossly carious, if root canal treatment has failed, if tooth is fractured or for orthodontic purposes. As long as the tooth is fully erupted, the operator will attempt to extract the tooth under local anaesthetic.

UNDER LOCAL ANAESTHETIC

Procedure
(1) Confirm consent with patient ensuring that all options and possible side effects have been discussed.
(2) Personal protective equipment is donned and the operator administers the local anaesthetic appropriate for the patient's medical history (see below – Local anaesthetics).
(3) After the local anaesthetic has taken effect the operator will refer to the radiograph and detach the periodontal ligament with an elevator of choice. The dental nurse will retract the soft tissues as required.
(4) The appropriate forceps will be used to remove the tooth from the socket, while the dental nurse supports the patient and monitors them for signs of distress.
(5) A pack is applied to the socket and when the operator is happy that bleeding is controlled, post-operative instructions will be given by the dental nurse (see Figure 6.3).
(6) If bleeding is not controlled with a pack (see Chapter 7, section Haemorrhage) a suture kit may be required. The operator will place and tie off the suture while the dental nurse retracts soft tissue and cuts the ends of the suture silk.

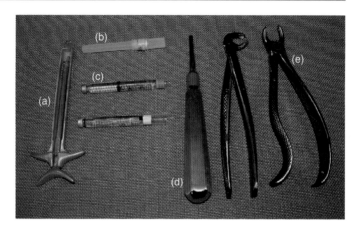

Fig. 6.1 Set-up for simple extraction under local anaesthetic. (a) Local anaesthetic (LA) syringe; (b) appropriate LA needle; (c) appropriate LA cartridge; (d) Coupland's osseous chisel; (e) appropriate extraction forceps. Additional equipment: Warwick-James elevators, Cryer's elevators, swabs, suture equipment.

UNDER SEDATION

Particularly anxious patients may elect to be treated under sedation. Patients who are sedated remain conscious but will be in a relaxed state. Sedation is achieved in three ways: orally, via inhalation and intravenously. Sedation should only be administered in practices which fulfil the General Dental Council guidelines.

Procedure

(1) Check that pre-operative instructions have been followed and that patient has an escort with them.

(2) Check patient's weight if necessary.

(3) Once the patient is seated and personal protective equipment has been provided for the team, the operator will administer the sedation while the dental nurse assists.

(4) The dental nurse will monitor the patient's well-being continuously throughout treatment.

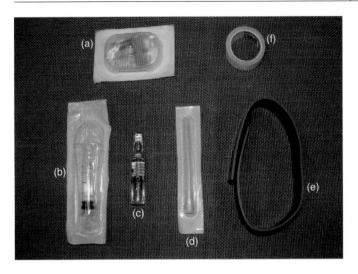

Fig. 6.2 Set-up and materials required for sedation. (a) Butterfly infusion set; (b) hypodermic syringe; (c) sedative drug ampoule; (d) hypodermic syringe; (e) tourniquet; (f) micropore tape. Additional equipment: cotton wool rolls.

(5) The operator then administers the local anaesthetic appropriate for the patient's medical history (see below – Local anaesthetics).

(6) After the local anaesthetic has taken effect the operator will refer to the radiograph and detach the periodontal ligament with an elevator of choice. The dental nurse will retract soft tissues as required.

(7) The appropriate forceps will be used to remove the tooth from the socket while the dental nurse supports the patient and monitors them for signs of distress.

(8) A pack is applied to the socket until the operator is happy that bleeding is controlled.

(9) If bleeding is not controlled with a pack (see Chapter 7, section Haemorrhage) a suture kit may be required. The operator will place and tie off the suture while the dental nurse retracts soft tissue and cuts the ends of the suture silk.

---

(1) You should expect some degree of pain after surgery. Purchase your usual painkillers from the chemist and take them as directed on the packaging.

(2) To avoid infection, you should rinse your mouth with hot salt water mouthwashes. Add one teaspoon of salt to a glass of hot water. This should start 6 hours after treatment and continue 4 times a day for 3–4 days.

(3) Avoid dislodging the clot in the socket. Do not undertake any vigorous exercise, don't smoke and try not to poke the area with your tongue.

(4) A soft diet may be advisable for the first day or so.

(5) As well as the mouthwashes, you should continue to clean your teeth as usual.

(6) If bleeding occurs, take a swab or clean handkerchief, dampen slightly and hold over the socket. Bite firmly for at least 15 minutes.

(7) If bleeding persists contact your dentist for advice.

Fig. 6.3 Post-operative instructions.

(10) The patient is then escorted to the recovery room by the dental nurse, who will remain and monitor the patient until recovered.

(11) The operator will make a decision about whether the patient is fit to leave and the escort will be called in.

(12) Post-operative instructions (Figure 6.3) are given verbally and in writing to the escort.

LOCAL ANAESTHETICS

Types of injection

Inferior dental nerve block
Given at the back of the mouth behind the last lower tooth. The tip of the needle is inserted near the nerve bundle and the analgesic is deposited around it.

Infiltration
Produces analgesia in a localised area. Analgesic solution injected into the tissue to affect nerve endings at the site, as opposed to applying to the nerve trunk.

Intra-ligamental
Produces analgesia for a single tooth. The needle is extremely fine and inserted down the side of the tooth into the periodontal ligament. The anaesthetic is injected under very high pressure.

Intra-osseous
This is only used when other methods of analgesia have failed. The gingiva and periosteum will have been made numb but there is still insufficient analgesia. A small hole is drilled into the alveolar bone adjacent to a tooth and the needle is inserted through the hole.

Topical/surface analgesia
Numbness can be produced by using a surface or topical analgesic. They are used prior to injection, and prior to impression taking and incising an abscess.

Contents of a local anaesthetic cartridge

	Xylotox, Xylocaine	**Citanest**
Local anaesthetic agent	Lidocaine 2%	Prilocaine 3%
Vasoconstrictor	Adrenaline 1 in 80 000	Felypressin
Other contents	Ringer's solution	Ringer's solution
	Antiseptic	Antiseptic
	Preservatives	Preservatives

The action of adrenaline is to constrict the blood vessels near the site of the injection. This keeps the local anaesthetic localised, increasing the depth and duration of the painlessness. Felypressin is a synthetic vasoconstrictor which is used in patients with certain medical conditions in which adrenaline is contraindicated.

Procedure

(1) Select the correct needle, cartridge and syringe for the patient and procedure. Check with the dentist.
(2) Break the seal on the needle and load into syringe.
(3) Remove cartridge from the sterile pack and load into the syringe.
(4) Check to see cartridge name and expiry date are showing. Also check to see if the solution is cloudy or contains sediment or crystals. If it does, discard immediately.
(5) Check to see if the fluid is flowing – do not remove the cover.
(6) Hand to the dentist with the needle cover in place.
(7) Do not leave the patient alone.

Local anaesthetic can sometimes be made more pleasant for the patient by warming the cartridge in warm water.

Patients must be warned before leaving the surgery not to eat or drink hot foods or liquids until the effect of the anaesthesia has worn off. It could cause burns and trauma.

Local anaesthetic syringes

Non-aspirating local anaesthetic syringe
Plunger has a flat end, which rests against the bung of the cartridge. Does not aspirate. Used for infiltration injections in the upper jaw.

Aspirating local anaesthetic syringe
Plunger has one or two claws at the end, which should be screwed into the bung of the cartridge. Allows for manual aspirating. Used for inferior dental block injections in the lower jaw.

Self-aspirating local anaesthetic syringe
Plunger is tapered to fit in the indentation of the specially adapted bung of the cartridges. Automatically aspirates when pressure on plunger is released. Used for inferior dental block injection in the lower jaw.

Minor Oral Surgery

7

Minor oral surgery is required in a range of treatments including complex extractions, apicectomy and biopsy. An aseptic technique should be used throughout the procedure to prevent transmission of infection directly into the blood stream.

COMPLEX EXTRACTIONS

Procedure

(1) Once the patient is seated in the dental chair, the dental nurse should confirm consent has been gained for the procedure and that the patient has followed any pre-operative instructions.

(2) Protective clothing, surgical gloves, mask and safety glasses (or visor) should be donned by the dental team and a surgical drape and safety glasses provided for the patient.

(3) Local anaesthetic is administered by the operator while the dental nurse reassures and monitors the patient as necessary.

(4) Once the anaesthetic has taken effect the dental nurse will be responsible for maintaining a clear field of vision by retracting the soft tissues and aspirating while the incision is made by the operator.

(5) A flap is raised and held away from the site with a periosteal elevator by the dental nurse.

(6) The operator will remove bone if necessary, using a surgical handpiece and bur while the dental nurse aspirates.

(7) Elevators and extraction forceps are passed to the operator as required by the dental nurse.

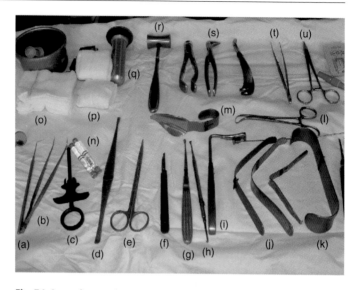

Fig. 7.1 Set-up for complex extractions under local anaesthetic. (a) Straight probe; (b) tweezers; (c) local anaesthetic syringe; (d) periosteal elevator; (e) tissue scissors; (f) scalpel handle and blade; (g) Laster's retractor; (h) Mitchell's trimmer; (i) rake retractor; (j) tongue retractors; (k) cheek retractor; (l) towel clip; (m) luxator; (n) local anaesthetic cartridges; (o) galley pot with saline and hypodermic syringe; (p) swabs; (q) handle cover; (r) mallet; (s) extraction forceps; (t) rat tooth tissue forceps; (u) needle holder. Additional equipment: mouth mirror, Coupland's osseous chisels, Yankaver's suction tip, Warwick-James elevators, Cryer's elevators, sutures and scissors, artery forceps.

(8) Throughout the procedure the dental nurse will monitor and reassure the patient and advise the operator if the patient appears in distress.

(9) Once the tooth (or teeth) has been removed the dental nurse will assist with the suturing of the flap and cutting the sutures as instructed by the operator.

(10) The dental nurse will then clean the patient and give them verbal and written versions of the post-operative instructions (see Figure 6.1).

(11) The operator will decide when the patient is well enough to leave the surgery.

APICECTOMY

Procedure

(1) Once the patient is seated in the dental chair, the dental nurse should confirm consent has been gained for the procedure and that the patient has followed any pre-operative instructions.

(2) Protective clothing, surgical gloves, mask and safety glasses (or visor) should be donned by the dental team and a surgical drape and safety glasses provided for the patient.

(3) Local anaesthetic is administered by the operator while the dental nurse reassures and monitors the patient if necessary.

(4) Once the anaesthetic has taken effect the dental nurse will be responsible for maintaining a clear field of vision by retracting the soft tissues and aspirating while the incision is made by the operator.

(5) A flap is raised and held away from the site with a periosteal elevator by the dental nurse.

(6) The operator will remove an area of bone overlying the apex of the tooth using a surgical handpiece and bur, and will remove all infected tissue using a curette or Mitchell's trimmer. The apex of the tooth is removed to allow a retrograde filling to be placed.

(7) The dental nurse will aspirate during this part of the procedure and, when requested, prepare the required filling material.

(8) Debris is aspirated by the dental nurse before the operator replaces the flap and places sutures.

(9) The dental nurse may assist with the placement of sutures, cutting them as instructed by the operator.

(10) The dental nurse will then clean the patient and give them verbal and written versions of the post-operative instructions (see Figure 6.3).

(11) The operator will decide when the patient is well enough to leave the surgery.

BIOPSY

Procedure

(1) Once the patient is seated in the dental chair, the dental nurse should confirm consent has been gained for the procedure and that the patient has followed any pre-operative instructions.

(2) Protective clothing, surgical gloves, mask and safety glasses (or visor) should be donned by the dental team and a surgical drape and safety glasses provided for the patient.

(3) Local anaesthetic is administered by the operator while the dental nurse reassures and monitors the patient if necessary.

(4) Once the anaesthetic has taken effect the dental nurse will be responsible for maintaining a clear field of vision by retracting the soft tissues and aspirating while the incision is made by the operator.

(5) Once the tissue sample has been removed it is placed, by the dental nurse, in a preserving solution in a sealed sample pot and sent to be tested with laboratory instructions.

(6) If necessary sutures are placed and the dental nurse may assist with this process, cutting the sutures as required.

(7) The dental nurse will then clean the patient and give them verbal and written versions of the post-operative instructions (see Figure 6.3).

(8) The operator will decide when the patient is well enough to leave the surgery.

HAEMORRHAGE

There are three types of haemorrhage that occur during and after a surgical procedure.

Primary haemorrhage

Primary haemorrhage is that which occurs at the time of the procedure and is caused by the cutting of blood vessels during the procedure. It is usually controlled by applying pressure to the area using a gauze pack. If pressure does not control the bleeding the operator may decide to place sutures.

Reactionary haemorrhage

Reactionary haemorrhage is caused usually within a few hours of the procedure and is caused by the clot being disturbed. This can be prevented by following the post-operative instructions, but if it does occur the patient should be advised to apply pressure to a clean gauze pack placed over the socket for 20 minutes. If this fails to control the bleeding the patient should be advised to attend the surgery where the operator may place a haemostatic dressing or sutures.

Secondary haemorrhage

Secondary haemorrhage is usually caused by an infection in the socket within a few days of the procedure having been carried out. The patient should return to the surgery immediately and have an antiseptic dressing placed. The operator may also decide to place sutures.

Orthodontics

8

The orthodontic branch of dentistry is concerned with the correction of malocclusion. Malocclusion occurs in different forms as does the treatment to improve it. Malocclusion can be improved merely by taking out certain teeth and allowing the adjacent teeth to drift and fill the space or the patient may be fitted with a removable or fixed appliance.

In all cases the patient must be motivated and have a high standard of oral hygiene.

REMOVABLE APPLIANCE

Procedure

Visit 1
(1) Having decided that the patient is suitable for removable appliance treatment, measurements, photographs and X-rays are taken and records kept in the patient's file.
(2) Impressions are taken of both jaws in alginate, which the dental nurse has prepared and placed in suitably sized trays.
(3) Study models are cast in the laboratory and the appliance designed by the operator. The lab technician then makes the appliance prior to the patient's next visit.

Visit 2
(1) The appliance is fitted in the patient's mouth and any adjustments made. Acrylic is trimmed using a laboratory handpiece and acrylic burs and any changes to the labial bow or Adams' clasps are made with the appropriate orthodontic pliers.

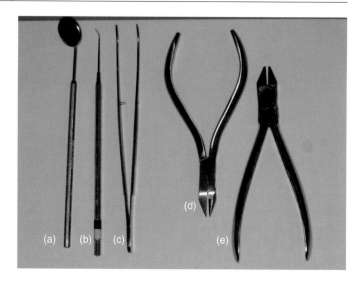

Fig. 8.1 Removable orthodontic appliance instrument tray. (a) Mirror; (b) probe; (c) tweezers; (d) light wire pliers; (e) Adams' universal pliers. Additional equipment: lab handpiece, acrylic trimming burs.

(2) Sometimes removable appliance treatment is supplemented with headgear. The headgear is also fitted at this appointment.

(3) The patient is given post-operative instructions by the dental nurse on the care of the appliance and maintaining oral hygiene.

(4) A review appointment is made to check progress.

FIXED APPLIANCE

Procedure

Visit 1

(1) Having decided that the patient is suitable for fixed appliance therapy, measurements, photographs and X-rays are taken and the records kept in the patient's file.

Orthodontic band

Orthodontic bracket

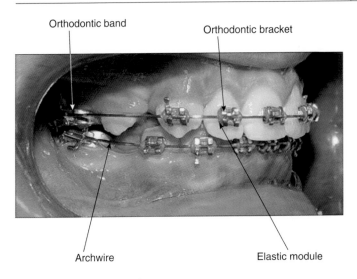

Archwire

Elastic module

Fig. 8.2 Fixed orthodontic appliance.

(2) Impressions are taken of both jaws in alginate, which the dental nurse has prepared and placed in suitably sized trays.
(3) Study models are cast in the laboratory and the appliance is designed by the operator.

Visit 2
(1) Orthodontic bands are selected and cemented onto the posterior teeth using a glass ionomer cement.
(2) Appropriate orthodontic brackets are selected, and the teeth to be bracketed are etched using an acid etchant placed in a dappen pot by the dental nurse.
(3) The teeth are then washed and dried with a 3-in-1 syringe while the dental nurse aspirates.
(4) The brackets are cemented to the teeth using a chemically cured composite cement.

8

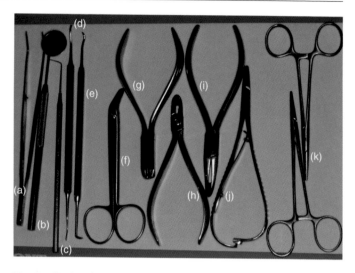

Fig. 8.3 Fixed orthodontic appliance instrument tray. (a) Tweezers; (b) mirror; (c) probe; (d) ligature tucker; (e) Mitchell's trimmer; (f) tape shears; (g) Matthews holders; (h) distal end cutter; (i) Weingart's pliers; (j) ligature cutters; (k) mosquito forceps. Additional equipment: cement, ligatures/elastic modules, archwires, orthodontic bands, orthodontic brackets.

(5) An archwire is selected and placed through the tubes on the orthodontic bands and across the front of the orthodontic brackets.

(6) The archwire is tied into the brackets using either elastic modules or ligatures which are passed by the dental nurse. Any elastics if needed are given to the patient.

(7) Oral hygiene advice and instructions about care of the appliance are given to the patient by the dental nurse, and a review appointment is made.

Note: the procedure described under Visit 2 may be carried out in more than one appointment.

Restorations

A restoration may be required for several reasons: caries, trauma, tooth wear or as part of a more extensive treatment plan. The material selected for the restoration will depend on the position of the restoration and why it is needed.

AMALGAM

Amalgam restorations are used in posterior cavities as the material is hardwearing and cheap. During the placement of an amalgam, care must be taken to ensure the risk of contact with mercury is kept to a minimum whether via the skin or by inhalation of the fumes emitted.

Procedure

(1) Once the patient is seated in the chair and personal protective equipment has been provided, local anaesthetic is administered according to the patient's medical history (see Chapter 3).

(2) The cavity is accessed using a high-speed handpiece and diamond bur while the dental nurse retracts soft tissue and aspirates fluid and debris.

(3) Caries is removed using a slow-speed handpiece and steel burs, again while the dental nurse retracts and aspirates.

(4) An excavator may be used at the base of the cavity to remove small amounts of caries before the cavity is shaped to retain the amalgam.

(5) If required the dental nurse will mix an appropriate lining material which is then placed into the cavity using a calcium hydroxide applicator or flat plastic.

(6) The amalgam is mixed using either an amalgamator or an encapsulated amalgam mixer and the mixed material is

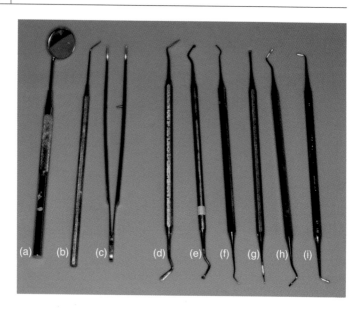

Fig. 9.1 Amalgam instrument tray. (a) Mirror; (b) probe; (c) tweezers; (d) flat plastic; (e) excavator; (f) excavator; (g) carver; (h) plugger; (i) pear-shaped burnisher. Additional equipment: matrix band, wedges, pin, amalgam carrier.

placed into a dappen dish before being handed to the operator in an amalgam carrier.

(7) Once the cavity is full, the operator will carve and burnish the amalgam using carvers and burnishers while the dental nurse aspirates any excess.

(8) The occlusion is checked using a piece of articulating paper placed by the dental nurse into a pair of Miller's forceps, and the amalgam is carved again to remove excess.

(9) Once the restoration is complete, the dental nurse may give the patient a mouthwash and post-operative instructions.

COMPOSITE

Composite is the material of choice for anterior teeth or for cosmetic reasons in posterior teeth. It is available in a range of shades and can be matched to the patient's tooth colour. Care must be taken when using the curing light and etchant material as each of these presents a hazard during use.

Procedure

(1) Once the patient is seated in the chair and personal protective equipment has been provided, local anaesthetic is administered according to the patient's medical history.

(2) Rubber dam can be placed at this stage, as composite materials are moisture sensitive.

(3) The cavity is accessed using a high-speed handpiece and diamond bur while the dental nurse retracts soft tissue and aspirates fluid and debris.

(4) Caries is removed using a slow-speed handpiece and steel burs, again whilst the dental nurse retracts and aspirates.

(5) Once the cavity is clean it is washed and dried using a 3-in-1 syringe while the dental nurse continues to aspirate.

(6) The enamel surfaces of the cavity are etched using an acid etchant and applicator, which is washed off after the appropriate amount of time while the dental nurse continues to aspirate.

(7) The cavity is dried thoroughly using the 3-in-1 syringe or a cotton wool pledget.

(8) Bonding agent is then applied to the dentine surfaces of the cavity and this is cured using the curing light. The light filter shield should be used during this process.

(9) Cellulose matrix may be placed if the mesial or distal surface of the tooth is involved.

(10) Composite material of an appropriate shade is placed incrementally into the cavity using a flat plastic and cured after placement of each increment.

(11) The restoration is then shaped and finished using finishing strips or abrasive discs and the occlusion checked using articulating paper held in Miller's forceps.

(12) The patient is given a mouthwash and postoperative instructions by the dental nurse.

9

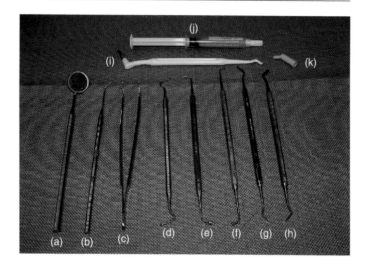

Fig. 9.2 Composite instrument tray. (a) Mouth mirror; (b) straight probe; (c) tweezers; (d) excavator; (e) plugger; (f) burnisher; (g) flat plastic; (h) Ward's carver; (i) applicator brush handle; (j) acid etchant; (k) composite material. Additional equipment: cellulose matrix strip, bonding agent, shade guide, curing light and shield.

> **TOP TIP**
> When selecting the appropriate shade for a patient try to use natural light – take the patient to a window if possible.

GLASS IONOMER

Glass ionomer is usually selected for restorations in children as it leaches fluoride and so helps strengthen the tooth against further decay. It is also often used in cervical cavities and is quick and simple to prepare. Glass ionomer bonds directly to both enamel and dentine so little cavity preparation is needed and less healthy tooth is destroyed.

Procedure

(1) Once the patient is seated in the chair and personal protective equipment has been provided, local anaesthetic is administered according to the patient's medical history.

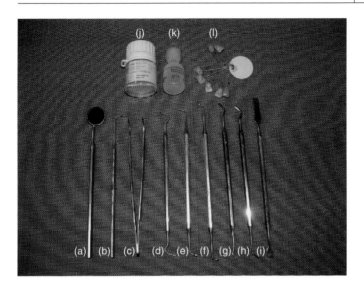

Fig. 9.3 Glass ionomer instrument tray. (a) Mouth mirror; (b) straight probe; (c) tweezers; (d) excavator; (e) plugger; (f) burnisher; (g) Ward's carver; (h) flat plastic; (i) mixing spatula; (j) glass ionomer powder; (k) distilled water; (l) shade guide.

(2) Rubber dam can be placed at this stage if required, as glass ionomer materials are moisture sensitive.

(3) The cavity is cleaned using a high-speed handpiece while the dental nurse retracts the soft tissue and aspirates fluid and debris.

(4) Caries is removed using a slow-speed handpiece and steel burs, again while the dental nurse retracts and aspirates.

(5) Once the cavity is washed and dried the dental nurse will prepare the appropriate amount and shade of glass ionomer, which is then inserted using a flat plastic.

(6) The restoration is shaped and if required, the occlusion checked using articulating paper held in Miller's forceps. Any debris is aspirated by the dental nurse.

(7) The patient is offered a mouthwash and given post-operative instructions by the dental nurse.

9

TEMPORARY FILLINGS

Temporary fillings may be placed in larger cavities or in a tooth in which root canal treatment is being carried out. They are intended to ensure that the tooth condition does not deteriorate between appointments, and should be replaced as soon as possible with a permanent restoration.

Procedure

(1) Once the patient is seated in the chair and personal protective equipment has been provided, local anaesthetic is administered according to the patient's medical history.

(2) The cavity is accessed using a high-speed handpiece and diamond bur while the dental nurse retracts the soft tissue and aspirates fluid and debris.

(3) Caries is removed using a slow-speed handpiece and steel burs, again while the dental nurse retracts and aspirates.

(4) Once the cavity is washed and dried the dental nurse will prepare the appropriate amount and shade of temporary filling material, which is then inserted using a flat plastic.

(5) The restoration is shaped and any debris is aspirated by the dental nurse.

(6) The patient is offered a mouthwash and given post-operative instructions by the dental nurse.

Crown and Bridge

10

Crowns are fitted on teeth for many reasons. Fractured teeth, grossly carious teeth and discoloured teeth can all be improved with a crown. There are many types of crown including porcelain jacket crown, porcelain bonded crown, post crown, full gold crown, and three quarter crown, but for all types of crown, the theory of crown preparation is the same. The teeth are trimmed down to make room for the structure of the crown to fit and impressions are taken so that the technician can make the desired crown in the laboratory.

PREPARATION

Procedure
(1) Once the patient is seated in the chair and personal protective equipment has been provided, local anaesthetic is administered according to the patient's medical history.
(2) An alginate impression is taken of the arch opposing the tooth to be crowned, and another alginate impression may be taken of the arch that will contain the crown to facilitate the creation of a temporary crown at the end of the procedure.
(3) The operator then, using handpiece and burs, will remove as much of the tooth structure as is required while the dental nurse aspirates.
(4) If a post crown is being fitted on an already root-filled tooth* the root canal is also prepared to allow room for the post.
(5) Once the tooth is prepared, a gingival retraction cord is inserted around the preparation, and if required a temporary post is fitted down the root canal.

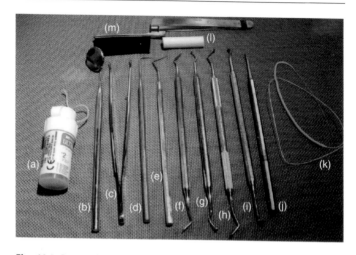

Fig. 10.1 Crown prep instrument tray. (a) Gingival retraction cord; (b) mirror; (c) tweezers; (d) probe; (e) periodontal probe; (f) flat plastic; (g) ball-ended burnisher; (h) pear-shaped burnisher; (i) Mitchell's trimmer; (j) enamel chisel; (k) superfloss; (l) cotton wool roll; (m) Miller's forceps. Additional equipment: high-speed handpiece, diamond burs, preformed temporary crown forms, temporary cement.

(6) A rubber-based impression material is prepared by the dental nurse and is used to take an impression of the prepared tooth by the operator.

(7) The impression is removed from the patient's mouth and the gingival retraction cord is removed using a pair of tweezers.

(8) A temporary crown can either be made using the alginate impression taken earlier or selected from a range of preformed temporary crown forms and cemented using a temporary crown cement.

(9) A shade is selected with the help of the dental nurse and the patient.

(10) A wax squash bite is taken using pink sheet wax and placed in a sealed bag along with the impressions taken earlier and the laboratory instruction sheet.

10

*If tooth is not already root filled then root canal treatment will be carried out first.

FIT

Procedure

(1) Once the patient is prepared, a local anaesthetic is given if required.
(2) The temporary crown is removed and excess cement removed from the surface of the tooth.
(3) The permanent crown is tried in and adjusted as necessary by the operator.
(4) Once the fit is satisfactory the crown is cemented with a permanent luting cement.
(5) The bite is then checked using articulating paper and adjusted as necessary by the operator.
(6) The patient is handed a mirror to check appearance and oral hygiene instructions are given.

Dentures

Dentures are removable prostheses given to patients to replace missing teeth. They can be used to replace a whole arch (complete dentures) or just a few teeth (partial dentures) and can be made from acrylic or cobalt chrome. Sometimes dentures can be made prior to the tooth being extracted and fitted on the day of the extraction (immediate dentures). The procedures for all of these types of denture are included in this chapter.

COMPLETE DENTURES

These are generally made in acrylic and constructed over five visits.

First appointment – primary impressions

(1) Once the patient is seated and personal protective equipment has been provided for the patient and the dental team, the operator will select an impression tray which best fits the patient's arch. This will be selected from the edentulous trays laid out by the dental nurse.

(2) Having found a tray that fits the patient the operator will be ready to take the alginate impression. The dental nurse will mix sufficient material according to manufacturer's instructions and load the tray before passing to the operator.

(3) While the impression is being taken the dental nurse will monitor the patient and reassure them. A bowl should be available in case the patient gags.

(4) Once the impression is set, it is removed from the patient's mouth and the dental nurse rinses it under running water to remove debris and places it in a disinfectant solution according to manufacturer's instructions.

(5) The impression is removed from the disinfectant, wrapped in damp gauze and placed in a bag ready for transport to the laboratory.

(6) The dental nurse will prepare a laboratory card for the operator to complete and this is then attached to the impression.

Second appointment – secondary impressions

(1) The dental nurse will ensure that the special trays are back from the laboratory and will prepare the surgery.

(2) The patient will then be brought in to the surgery and provided with personal protective equipment.

(3) The operator will try-in the tray to check the fit and extend using greenstick composition and a Bunsen burner if required.

(4) The dental nurse will place Vaseline (petroleum jelly) around the patient's lips and prepare the zinc oxide and eugenol impression paste for loading into the tray before handing to the operator.

(5) Once the impression material is set, the dental nurse will rinse and disinfect the impressions and place them into a bag ready for transport to the laboratory. The operator will update the laboratory card.

(6) The dental nurse will assist the patient in cleaning their face before they leave the surgery.

Third appointment – jaw relations

(1) The surgery is prepared for recording jaw relations and the dental nurse will retrieve the wax rims which have been returned from the laboratory.

(2) The operator will measure the freeway space using a Willis bite gauge while the dental nurse records the measurements in the patient's notes.

(3) Location grooves will be cut into each wax rim by the operator and the dental nurse will prepare the zinc oxide and eugenol impression paste and pass to the operator for the jaw relationship to be checked.

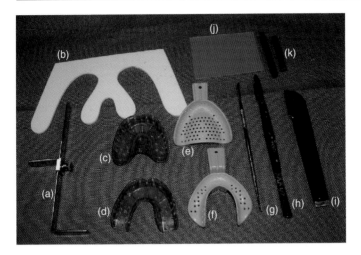

Fig. 11.1 Instrument tray for bite registration. (a) Willis bite gauge; (b) Fox's occlusal plane guide; (c) upper dentate impression tray; (d) lower dentate impression tray; (e) lower edentulous impression tray; (f) lower edentulous impression tray; (g) Le Cron's carver; (h) wax knife; (i) plaster knife; (j) pink sheet wax; (k) composition stick. Additional equipment: alginate, Bunsen burner, handpiece and acrylic burs, articulating paper, Miller's forceps.

(4) Once set, the wax rims are disinfected and the dental nurse will assist with taking the shade for the try-in stage.
(5) The patient is again assisted to clean their face and given an appointment for the next visit.

Fourth appointment – wax try-in
(1) Once the surgery has been prepared and the patient and dental team have been provided with personal protective equipment, the patient will be asked to try-in the wax dentures.
(2) The operator will check the freeway space and the occlusal registration and the patient will be asked if they are happy with the appearance of the teeth. Any alterations are made at this stage.

Fifth appointment – fit

(1) Once the surgery has been prepared and the patient and dental team have been provided with personal protective equipment, the patient will be asked to try on the new dentures.

(2) The operator will check the occlusion using articulating paper and any sore spots will be eased using a laboratory handpiece and acrylic burs. The freeway space is checked again at this stage.

(3) The dental nurse will then give the patient instructions about caring for their dentures (see p. 103) and a review appointment is made.

PARTIAL DENTURES

Partial dentures are usually constructed in cobalt chrome and any restorative treatment, periodontal treatment and extractions required should always be carried out beforehand.

First appointment – primary impressions

(1) Once the patient is seated and personal protective equipment has been provided for the patient and the dental team, the operator will select an impression tray which best fits the patient's arch. This will be selected from the dentate trays laid out by the dental nurse.

(2) Having found a tray that fits the patient the operator will be ready to take the alginate impression. The dental nurse will mix sufficient material according to manufacturer's instructions and load the tray before passing to the operator.

(3) During the taking of the impression the dental nurse monitors the patient and reassures them. A bowl should be available in case the patient gags.

(4) Once the impression is set it is removed from the patient's mouth, and the dental nurse rinses it under running water to remove debris and places it in a disinfectant solution according to manufacturer's instructions.

(5) The impression is removed from the disinfectant, wrapped in damp gauze and placed in a bag ready for transport to the laboratory.

(6) The dental nurse will prepare a laboratory card for the operator to complete and this is then attached to the impression.

Second appointment – tooth preps and secondary impressions

(1) The spaced special trays should be retrieved from the laboratory and the surgery prepared before the patient is brought in and given personal protective equipment. Personal protective equipment is also provided for the dental team.

(2) The operator may need to cut rest seats in the enamel of the teeth using a high-speed handpiece and appropriate burs according to the framework design.

(3) A rubber-based material is prepared by the dental nurse and loaded into the special tray before passing to the operator. On removal from the mouth the dental nurse rinses and disinfects the impression before placing in a bag and attaching the updated lab card.

Third appointment – try-in framework and jaw relations

(1) The chrome framework with wax rims should be retrieved from the laboratory and the surgery prepared before the patient is brought in and given personal protective equipment. Personal protective equipment is also provided for the dental team.

(2) The chrome framework is tried in and any minor adjustments are made by the operator.

(3) The wax rims are softened and the patient is asked to bite into the softened wax to show the occlusal registration. The dental nurse monitors and reassures the patient throughout.

(4) If posterior teeth are missing zinc oxide and eugenol impressions are taken of the free-end saddle. The dental nurse places Vaseline (petroleum jelly) around the patient's mouth before mixing the impression material and passing to the dentist to place in the free-end saddle.

(5) The dental nurse will disinfect the impression on removal from the mouth and assist in taking the shade of teeth for the try-in stage.

Fourth appointment – try-in

(1) The chrome framework with teeth set in wax should be retrieved from the laboratory and the surgery prepared before the patient is brought in and given personal protective equipment. Personal protective equipment is provided for the dental team.

(2) The patient will be asked to try in the framework again and the tooth position checked.

(3) The appearance of the denture is checked with the patient and any alterations are made at this stage

Fifth appointment – fit

(1) The denture should be retrieved from the laboratory and the surgery prepared before the patient is brought in and given personal protective equipment. Personal protective equipment is also provided for the dental team.

(2) The patient is given the new denture to try in and the operator will check the occlusion and the appearance.

(3) The patient will be shown by the operator how to insert and remove the denture safely, and the dental nurse will give denture care instructions (see p. 103).

(4) The patient is given a date for a review appointment.

Immediate dentures

Immediate dentures are used when a patient has some existing teeth which need extracting and the denture is fitted the same day as the extractions.

Immediate dentures are made in exactly the same way as either complete or partial acrylic dentures (depending on whether the patient will have any teeth remaining) until the try-in stage. Because the tooth to be replaced is still *in situ* a try-in is not possible.

Fourth appointment – fit and extraction

(1) The chrome framework with teeth set in wax should be retrieved from the laboratory and the surgery prepared before the patient is brought in and given personal protective

equipment. Personal protective equipment is also provided for the dental team.

(2) Extractions are carried out (see Chapter 6).

(3) The denture is fitted as above with alterations being kept to a minimum.

(4) The dental nurse monitors and reassures the patient throughout and makes the patient an appointment for the following day so that alterations can be made to the denture.

DENTURE CARE

- Clean dentures after every meal using soap and a toothbrush. You should not use toothpaste as it is too abrasive and your normal toothbrush is usually sufficient. Denture brushes tend to be too large and do not clean the fitting surface effectively. They are only good if the patient has difficulty in holding a brush as denture brushes often have larger handles.

- When cleaning dentures always clean them over a bowl of water in case you drop them. This way they will not break and shatter in the sink.

- When cleaning partial dentures that have clasps ensure you do not bend or snap the clasps.

- Do not clean or immerse chrome cobalt dentures in hypochlorite as it stains and discolours them.

- Take out dentures at night and store in cold water. This gives the tissues time to breathe. Never store in hot water as this makes the denture go white.

- If you wish to use a denture cleaner try to use it once a week only – if used too often they bleach the acrylic.

- If you have denture-related stomatitis, your denture **should** be cleaned thoroughly in hypochlorite and stored in diluted hypochlorite at night.

RELINING A COMPLETE DENTURE

After teeth are extracted the alveolar bone resorbs or shrinks causing dentures to become loose. If the patient is pleased with the appearance and the occlusion of the denture, but is unhappy with the fit, a permanent reline may be the answer. A permanent reline involves only two visits for the patient.

Impressions

(1) The surgery is prepared before the patient is brought in and given personal protective equipment. Personal protective equipment is also provided for the dental team.

(2) The operator will prepare the denture to be relined so that an impression can be taken with it.

(3) The dental nurse will place Vaseline around the patient's mouth and mix the zinc oxide and eugenol impression material and pass to the operator who will place it in the patient's mouth.

(4) The opposing denture is also put in the mouth and the patient is asked to bite.

(5) The dental nurse will then disinfect the impression and prepare for transport to the laboratory.

(6) Once the patient is clean, they are given an appointment for the following day.

Fit

See "Complete dentures, Fifth appointment – Fit" above.

Dental Implants

The provision of dental implants requires the
dental nurse to have the necessary competencies
to assist the clinician and to understand the needs
of the patient.

WHAT ARE DENTAL IMPLANTS?

Dental implants replace missing teeth. A metal 'rod', usually
made of titanium, is inserted into the jawbone to replace the
missing tooth root. The rod is then used to support a replacement
tooth, this could be a crown, part of a bridge or a denture.

WHO CAN HAVE DENTAL IMPLANTS?

A **pre-assessment** of the patient is carried out where consideration will be given to the following general issues before the full
examination and assessment take place:

- Is the patient a heavy smoker?
- Does the patient drink alcohol excessively?
- Does the patient's medical condition contraindicate treatment,
  e.g. uncontrolled diabetes?
- Are the patient's expectations of the final result realistic?
- What is the condition of the patient's oral health?
- Is the patient going to be able to maintain good oral health
  when treatment is completed?

If any of the responses to these questions show that the success
of the treatment may be detrimentally affected, the patient may
not be recommended for treatment or treatment may be deferred
until a later date.

THE DENTAL NURSE'S ROLE IN THE PRE-ASSESSMENT STAGE
- ❏ Understand the needs of the patient and respect their right to confidentiality.
- ❏ Provide support to the dentist on general and oral health advice given.
- ❏ Give patient written information to take away with them (leaflets).
- ❏ Make valid, accurate, reliable, current and sufficient notes and present to dentist for verification.

THE STAGES OF DENTAL IMPLANT TREATMENT
(1) Clinical assessment
(2) Treatment planning
(3) Surgical placement of implant fixtures
(4) Impressions
(5) Fitting of implant restorations

Stage 3 may be carried out by an implantologist, and stages 4 and 5 by a prosthodontist, however, in some cases these may be one and the same.

Note: Universal cross-infection control procedures must be adopted throughout all stages.

STAGE 1 – CLINICAL ASSESSMENT
Once the dentist has determined from the results of the pre-assessment that the patient is suitable to be assessed for dental implants a more detailed assessment and examination of the oral cavity and anatomical structures is carried out.

The dental nurse's role in clinical assessment
- ❏ Have patient record card ready.
- ❏ Lay out relevant X-rays (direct exposure only if qualified to do so).
- ❏ Prepare patient for orthopantomogram (OPG) if required.
- ❏ Prepare impression material for preliminary study models.
- ❏ Lay out face measuring instruments.
- ❏ Prepare and take photographs (if competent to do so).

❑ Make valid, accurate, reliable, current and sufficient notes and present to dentist for verification.

STAGE 2 – TREATMENT PLANNING

The dentist will decide on the most appropriate treatment plan which is specific to the individual patient. This will include a timetable of treatment, the cost of the treatment, the number of implants required and the prosthesis most suitable for this patient.

The dental nurse's role in treatment planning

❑ Make available **all** records relating to the patient as listed in Stage 1.
❑ Assist the dentist with planning as necessary.
❑ Prepare a detailed costing for the patient.
❑ Prepare impression materials for the construction of the temporary prosthesis and surgical stent. Complete laboratory ticket (if applicable).
❑ Provide the patient with pre-operative instructions in order to prepare for Stage 3:
  –wear loose comfortable clothing;
  –have a light meal (a soft diet may be recommended post-operatively, therefore the patient may want to shop prior to appointment);
  –no face make-up or nail enamel to be worn;
  –antibiotics and analgesics may be prescribed, therefore patient may want to arrange to be escorted from the surgery and cared for at home.
❑ Confirm the patient's understanding of all instructions and obtain their signature of consent to the treatment.
❑ Make valid, accurate, reliable, current and sufficient notes and present to dentist for verification.
❑ Inform the patient of the next appointment.

STAGE 3 – SURGICAL PLACEMENT OF IMPLANT FIXTURES

An operating room or a well-prepared dental surgery is suitable for this procedure. If using the latter it must be cleared, cleaned and disinfected to simulate an operating theatre.

The placement of the implant fixture and healing abutment may be split into two stages:

One stage – implant and abutment placed for soft tissue healing

or

Two stage – in the first surgical procedure the implant and screw cover are placed (both under the gum line) with nothing showing above, only sutures. During the second procedure, the cover screw is removed and the healing abutment placed above the gum to encourage soft tissue healing.

The dental nurse's role in surgical placement of implant fixtures

For large or complex cases the ideal staffing situation would consist of two sterile dental nurses (one to retract and or aspirate, the second to pass sterile instruments and change the drills in the correct sequence) and one non-sterile dental nurse for each surgeon (clinician). The non-sterile dental nurse helps set up the surgery, tie gowns, open packages as and when required, place items in reach of surgeon or sterile dental nurse and keep a written note of what has been used. In most cases there are three people in attendance: surgeon (clinician), sterile dental nurse and non-sterile dental nurse. Often there are only two people available to undertake the various roles: the surgeon and sterile dental nurse, in this case the surgeon would help set up the surgery and the sterile dental nurse would de-glove to open components or do any duties out of the operating zone and then put on new sterile gloves to return to the chairside.

Preparation – room, equipment and instruments

(1) Make available **all** records relating to the patient as listed in Stage 1 (place in non-sterile zone).
(2) Check temporary restoration and surgical stent has arrived from laboratory (if applicable).
(3) Check suction filters and aspirator tubes.
(4) Place disposable plastic sheaths on all equipment or sterile covers.

Lay out the following items:

❏ surgical drilling motor and sterile handpiece;
❏ sterile irrigation equipment and sterile saline with back-up syringe;
❏ sterile suction tubes, large for back of the mouth (or 'main aspiration') and finer tube for operating site;
❏ sterile drapes on work surfaces and stands;
❏ sterile tubing covers;
❏ anaesthetic and syringe and additional sterile syringe if top-up required during operation;
❏ sterile gauze, mirror, probe, tweezers and small bowl for bone particles;
❏ drill/instrument organiser kit – drill side (Figure 12.1);
❏ drill/instrument organiser kit – instrument side (Figure 12.2).

Lay out minor oral surgery instrument kit: scalpels, cheek retractors, elevators, scissors–dissecting/suture, forceps (if teeth are being extracted) and artery forceps (see Figure 7.1).

Note: The above are suggested items and may not be used by all clinicians/surgeons in all cases.

Patient items:
❏ sterile drapes;
❏ cap;
❏ eye protection;
❏ antiseptic mouth rinse;
❏ long clamps and bowl of chlorhexidine solution to clean patient's face and gauze swabs.

The patient may be fully covered with a drape where only the face is visible, if a non-sterile dental nurse is present they will put the patient's cap and eye protection on but the sterile dental nurse will place the sterile drape around the patient.

Staff items:
❏ cap;
❏ mask;
❏ eye protection;

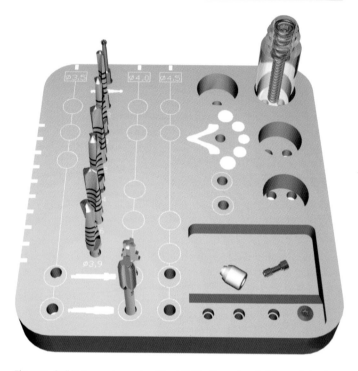

Fig. 12.1 Drill/instrument organiser kit – drill side. (Reproduced with permission from Neoss Ltd.)

❏ sterile gloves (non-sterile dental nurse will need additional gloves to clear away);
❏ sterile gowns.

Before commencing effective hand hygiene technique must be carried out by all staff (see Figure 2.1) and the dental nurse must confirm that the patient has followed pre-operative instructions.

During the procedure (the actual duties will depend on how many dental nurses are present as described under 'The dental nurse's role' at the start of Stage 3):

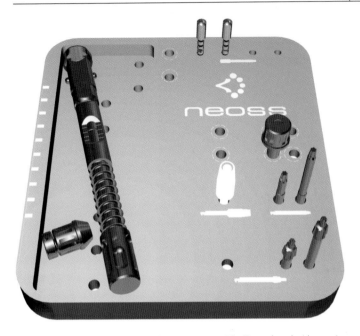

Fig. 12.2 Drill/instrument organiser kit – instrument side. (Reproduced with permission from Neoss Ltd.)

❏ observe patient throughout, check for signs of distress, notify surgeon immediately;
❏ aspirate at the back of the mouth and site of operation;
❏ retract flap tissue;
❏ assist with irrigation technique for bone preparation;
❏ change drills and pass instruments;
❏ open packages and place in reach of surgeon;
❏ ensure all packages and components used are accounted for and listed;
❏ prepare luting cement for temporary crown/bridge (if applicable) or reline material if the denture is temporary;
❏ X-ray films in plastic outer packaging are disinfected prior to being taken (not all surgeons take X-rays at this stage);

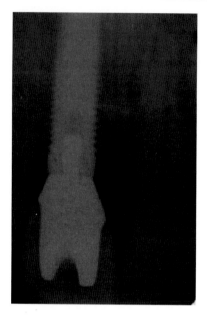

Fig. 12.3 Radiograph with implant fixture in place. (Reproduced with permission from Neoss Ltd.)

❑ assist surgeon to take X-ray (if competent to do so) (Figure 12.3);
❑ make valid, accurate, reliable, current and sufficient notes and present to surgeon for verification.

Post-operative patient care

The dental nurse will instruct the patient on how to care for the abutment and temporary prosthesis at home. This should include:

❑ cleaning with a non-abrasive toothpaste;
❑ using a soft-bristle toothbrush;
❑ rinsing with a non-acidic mouth wash at least once a day;
❑ if natural teeth are present follow usual oral hygiene regimen;

❏ inform that the surgeon/clinician or dental nurse will telephone the patient a few hours after the procedure to check on
their oral and general health;
❏ provide emergency telephone number;
❏ inform the patient of the next appointment.

Cleaning and sterilisation procedures

Always follow the manufacturer's instructions and guidelines
when carrying out this procedure. However, general rules apply
as for all other equipment.

❏ Check that instruments and drills are suitable to be reused
and disposed of safely if not.
❏ All other instruments, drills and the drill/instrument organiser should be hand cleaned under running water with a
brush and detergent as recommended by the manufacturer,
then rinsed clean.
❏ Place in ultrasonic bath. When cycle is complete, rinse under
running water and dry instruments (non-lint cloth).
❏ Place instruments in a sterilisation pouch and autoclave
(instruments used for implants should be placed in a vacuum
autoclave where possible).
❏ Implant drills, etc. placed in organiser must be dry before
returning to the storage area.
❏ Remove all drapes, disposable shields and carry out usual
decontamination procedures as described in Chapters 1
and 2.
❏ Ensure replacement instruments and drills are reordered
immediately.

STAGE 4 – IMPRESSIONS (TAKEN WHEN HEALING HAS COMPLETED)
❏ Make available **all** records relating to the patient as listed in
Stage 1.
❏ Lay out appropriate equipment and instruments (exact items
will depend on whether a healing abutment has been used or
the permanent abutment was inserted at Stage 3).
❏ Aspirate and assist surgeon/clinician removing the tempo-
rary healing abutments.

❏ Prepare impression materials for construction of permanent prosthesis and complete laboratory ticket (impression may also be taken to have the permanent customised abutment constructed).
❏ Make valid, accurate, reliable, current and sufficient notes and present to surgeon/clinician for verification.
❏ Inform patient about next appointment.

STAGE 5 – FITTING OF IMPLANT RESTORATIONS
❏ Check permanent restoration has arrived from laboratory.
❏ Make available **all** records relating to the patient as listed in Stage 1.
❏ Lay out appropriate equipment and instruments.
❏ Provide chairside assistance by aspirating, passing instruments/equipment and preparing luting cement for permanent restoration.
❏ Provide mirror for patient and confirm acceptance.
❏ Make valid, accurate, reliable, current and sufficient notes and present to dentist for verification.

POST-OPERATIVE PATIENT CARE
Maintenance of the prosthesis must be clearly explained to the patient:

❏ clean thoroughly around the restorations as if cleaning natural teeth;
❏ keep regular appointments for review of oral health including soft tissue, bone levels and prosthesis;
❏ attend regular hygienist appointments.

Make valid, accurate, reliable, current and sufficient notes and present to dentist for verification.

TOP TIPS
1. Strict cross-infection control procedures must be adopted at all times, particularly during surgical procedures. Where both sterile and non-sterile dental nurses are in

attendance each person must stay within their working zone and only carry out the duties assigned to them.

2. Pay particular attention to packaging symbols, which state if an item is sterile or non-sterile, single-use only (see Figure 2.4), expiry date, lot/batch number and any other issues which require special attention.

3. The dental nurse must ensure dental records are valid, accurate, reliable, current and sufficient and presented to the dentist for verification. All details relating to every stage of the treatment must be recorded including the equipment used and specific details about lot/batch numbers.

4. Dental nurses should ensure they are competent to assist during dental implant procedures. To achieve competence they may have to attend a training course organised by the implant supply company or attain a qualification as part of their continuing professional development.

LINKS TO OTHER CHAPTERS

- Chapter 4 – Dental Radiography.
- Chapter 7 – Minor Oral Surgery.

Patient Care and Management 13

> The way in which you use your verbal and non-verbal communication skills will affect your ability to provide effective patient care and support.

It is likely that one of the reasons you became a dental nurse is that you are interested in people. You may be the sort of person friends contact to talk over a problem and you may have appreciated someone listening to your concerns. This interest in people will be an advantage in your role and help you to support patients, and their families, carers, managers and colleagues.

In this chapter the main topics will be:

- Communicating with patients, helping them understand important aspects of their treatment and motivating them to improve their oral health
- Techniques for enhancing your communication skills
- Monitoring patients in the surgery
- Dealing with patients' complaints

Caring for patients, whether in the surgery or waiting room, includes understanding the needs of each individual, assessing how best to communicate information and provide support concerning their dental treatment. There are many ways to impart meaning and messages to others; it isn't just what you say that creates an impression. How you express the words, what you wear, how you stand, behave, listen and respond will affect the impact you have on the patients. It is easy to communicate messages that we don't intend to give. For example a receptionist could be welcoming a new patient to the practice with a smile, while sitting behind a desk (a barrier) with her arms crossed (another barrier) looking at her watch because the dentist is

For the Dental Nurse	For the patients
Enables you to obtain and give information that is relevant to the patient's dental care and well-being	Enables the patient to feel secure and respected at times when they are nervous and feel vulnerable – they feel able to express their needs, concerns and wishes
Having gained the trust and understanding of a patient you are able to form a relationship and be able to support them in making the most of the resources available	Patients feel able to maintain their sense of personal identity – co-operation and partnership is needed in open supportive communication

Fig. 13.1 The benefits of effective communication.

running late. Unfortunately the words and the smile may not be enough to convince the patient that the message is genuine. Experiments have shown that verbal communication is not the most effective method of expressing ourselves – 55% is communicated non-verbally. Equally it is easy for us to make judgements about patients and colleagues using our prejudices.

METHODS OF COMMUNICATION (Figure 13.1)

Verbal communication

Effective verbal communication involves speaking and listening to others. In dentistry our interactions may include conversations about: making appointments, obtaining confidential information/consent, giving specific instructions, promotion of an effective oral health regimen and dealing with problems or dental emergencies.

It is helpful to take the opportunity to observe the patient and learn from them, you may be able to respond to individuals better by observing:

• Is the person happy or sad?
• What is the person's attitude to others and to his or her surroundings?
• Is the person anxious or tense?
• Can the person see?

- Can the person hear?
- Can the person talk or is signing used?

An unhappy patient may have issues which they will consider far more serious than listening to your oral health advice. To continue to give the advice would be inappropriate if the patient is worried about losing their job, for instance. It is often easier to identify and satisfy patients with physical needs whereas emotional needs are more difficult to satisfy. Talking about your own feelings can sometimes help a patient to come to terms with a situation. When a patient relates to you sufficiently to 'open up', be ready to listen. A good listener hears what the patient says and interprets what the person means. At an appropriate point in the conversation you can check with the person whether you have understood everything by recalling what they have said. This is called reflective listening, it reassures you that you have interpreted the correct messages and shows to the patient that you are listening and are genuinely concerned. As you listen you will develop empathy, when you understand a person's feelings and are able to put yourself in their position.

It is important to respect the trust the patient has shown you, be discreet but seek help when necessary.

Relating to individuals
There are a number of skills which will help you to communicate effectively:

- take the opportunity to initiate a conversation;
- observe the person's behaviour;
- listen actively and reflectively;
- show empathy;
- know when to keep quiet;
- know how to 'read' and use non-verbal communication;
- respect people as individuals.

If you speak in a normal calm and controlled tone you often find that the listener will reflect your style and remain calm. If we talk in an aggressive or excitable tone the listener may be inclined to follow our example. You can try this out by asking a colleague

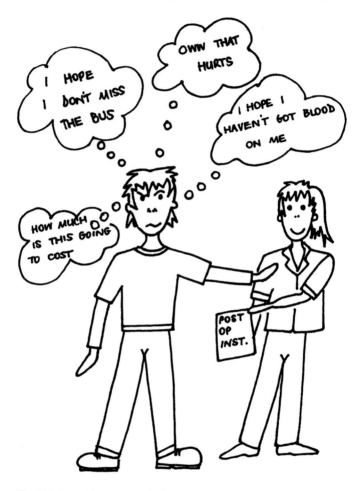

Fig. 13.2 Some information can be best passed on to patients in writing.

to speak to you using a normal tone and then switching to a more aggressive tone. See how it feels to be on the receiving end!

Always give the person you are speaking to priority over a phone call, failure to do this makes the patient feel unimportant and gives them the impression that you are not interested in them; you can always pick up a message on the answer phone afterwards. When you want to put across some oral health advice it is important to give the key points early on in the conversation. Don't be afraid to repeat these key points at the end. Using pictures, drawing a clear diagram or giving handouts will often help the patient to memorise information (Figure 13.2). Videos/ DVDs selected especially to suit the patient can be good, but it is important to make sure that there is not too much dental jargon.

Non-verbal communication
An understanding and awareness of non-verbal communication or body language will give you some insight and skill in your role as a dental nurse – not just where patients are concerned, communicating with colleagues is just as important. Research has shown that more human communication takes place by the use of:

- Facial expression – one of the most significant signs is a smile. Smiling shows warmth and openness.
- Gaze and eye contact – gaze as distinct from a casual glance tends to convey an interest which has the effect of increasing the other person's awareness of you. Eye contact is a fundamental part of getting on well with people. However, others may find it difficult to return your gaze, they may be shy, nervous or timid. Some cultures teach that it is impolite to look directly at people.
- Gestures and body movements – gesticulations, head movements all add emphasis to what we are saying, adding to the impression we create. Tilting your head to one side shows that you are actively listening while nodding the head slowly suggests that you are listening and wish the other person to continue. Hand shakes can give rise to misunderstanding, gestures have different meanings in different countries and

cultures. Drumming fingers, jangling keys and twiddling thumbs implies impatience. Rubbing your nose or eyes may be interpreted as a barrier or form of avoidance. If a person tells you they understand what you mean while scratching their head they may not actually understand at all.

- Body postures – stretching back in your chair away from a person sends a message that you are distant and don't care, while leaning forward, nodding and saying 'yes' reinforces your interest in that person. You may come across someone sitting in the waiting room with their arms crossed, this could mean that the person is acting defensively.
- Body contact – this is a difficult area and you need to be confident and assess the likely response of the person before you act. Occasionally a hand on the shoulder or arm can be very reassuring especially with children. Everyone has their own personal space where they feel comfortable, there are a number of zones.

Intimate zone	15–46 cm (6–18 inches)
Personal zone	0.5–1.2 m (18–48 inches)
Social zone	1.2–3.5 m (4–12 feet)
Public zone	3.5 m plus (12 feet plus)

BARRIERS TO COMMUNICATION

Your ability to get your message across effectively can be hindered by a number of barriers. You will need to recognise barriers to your own communication and learn how to overcome them.

- **Language** – As a multi-ethnic society, the UK has many citizens whose first language is not English and who find English difficult to understand. Many native speakers of English also find complicated medical terms and notices difficult to understand.
- **Culture** – We often take it for granted that another person's culture is similar to our own, yet in the UK there are many cultural differences within the population.

DISABILITY – PATIENTS WHO NEED SPECIAL CARE
One definition of disability is: the loss or limitation of opportunities to take part in normal life of the community on an equal level with others due to a physical and social barrier. In the UK 1 in 8 of the population is disabled. Two-thirds of the people with disabilities in the UK are over the age of 65 years. In 1995 the **Disability Discrimination Act** was introduced with far-reaching consequences; by 2004 there was a requirement for dental practices to provide reasonable access and communication aids to people with disabilities.

It is often difficult for disabled patients to receive the special care they need as there is often limited access to the surgery, they may have challenging behaviour and find it difficult to communicate and there may not be staff available who have the necessary training and experience. Dental surgeries need to be able to accommodate wheelchairs and walking frames. Alternatively, a domiciliary visit may be easier to manage although there are significant health and safety issues to consider. The British Society for Disability and Oral Health (www.bsdh.org.uk) has drawn up guidelines for dental care.

If you are interested in learning more about special care dental nursing, information is available in the book *Advanced Dental Nursing* (see references at the end of the chapter) or contact the National Examining Board for Dental Nurses, which will be able to give information on courses leading to their qualification – the Certificate in Special Care Dentistry.

AT THE CHAIRSIDE
Chairside manner matters because it indicates to patients whether they can trust us. A good manner with patients develops in the light of each patient's individual needs. It is grounded in the timeless virtues of honesty, humour and humility – explanations reduce anxiety.

You could use this checklist to make sure that you are doing all you can to instil confidence in your patients.

Checklist
❏ Friendly greeting – address the patients using their correct name (they may not always wish you to use their first name).

❏ Be on time – if you are unavoidably delayed explain to the patient giving a reason and give them an estimated new time.

❏ Use your interpersonal skills to develop empathy.

❏ Explain the practice policies so the patient understands from the start what to expect.

❏ Be optimistic – use positive language.

❏ Be open and consistent – listen carefully.

❏ Give information which is acceptable to the patient and check their understanding.

❏ Prioritise information – don't overload. Always give an opportunity to ask questions.

❏ Take the opportunity to praise even if progress is small.

❏ Use constructive feedback to reinforce behaviour.

THE PATIENT'S CHARTER

In the Patient's Charter the government has set out the patient's rights and standards of service which they should expect to be delivered in statutory National Health Service (NHS) health and social care environments.

Some examples of the standards
Every patient has the right to:

• access to their health records and knowledge that everyone working in the NHS is under a legal responsibility to keep them confidential;

• have any complaint about the NHS service investigated and have a quick, full, written reply;

• change their general practitioner/general dental practitioner easily and quickly;

• expect all staff they meet to wear a name badge.

PATIENT MONITORING

As a dental care professional it is part of the dental nurse's responsibility to be aware of the patient's well-being throughout their visit to the surgery. Being able to observe the patient and understand the significance of their conduct could be a valuable resource in preventing a medical emergency or disagreement with an anxious patient.

Signs to look for:

- over talkative;
- breathless;
- sweating;
- fidgeting;
- pallor.

CLINICAL MONITORING AT THE CHAIRSIDE

Checking respiration and pulse rates throughout treatment will give an indication of the patient's well-being.

- Respiration rate – assess the number of breaths for 30 seconds and then double the number to calculate the rate per minute which should be between 15 and 18. For a baby about 1 year old the rate would be about 24 breaths a minute.
- Pulse rate – use two fingers to feel the carotid pulse in the neck between the trachea (windpipe) and the large muscle in the neck – the rate in a resting adult is about 72 beats per minute.
- Skin colour – if the person has pale mucosae and perspiration on their forehead or upper lip then stop treatment and check the patient is feeling all right. A high colour may mean that the person is feverish or too hot.

PATIENT COMPLAINTS

Even the most successful dental practices receive complaints from patients. The way the complaint is managed will make the difference between causing a major disruption to the practice upsetting other patients and staff in the vicinity to using the complaint in a constructive way to improve the practice procedures.

A genuine patient complaint gives you an insight into how patients see the service you provide. Figure 13.3 can be a useful approach when dealing with a complaint.

It may be helpful to ask yourself why the patient was angry – and see what you could do to help them. The difficulty may not

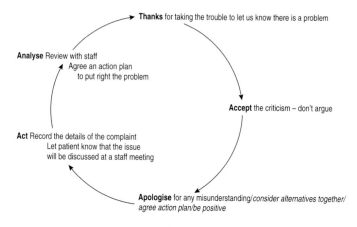

Fig. 13.3 An approach for dealing with patient complaints.

be related to the way they have been treated at the surgery. The General Dental Council's guidance document *Principles of Complaint Handling* explains the procedure it follows if a patient refers a complaint to the Council.

GIVING ORAL HEALTH ADVICE

Many practices have an area where patients can receive oral health advice (preventive dental care unit) on a one-to-one basis or sometimes in small groups. This is an important area as it is non-threatening to the patient, removing them from the surgery environment, encouraging them to participate and ask questions. A few well-designed posters and handouts will help to put across the message. The advice can be given by any member of the team who has sufficient knowledge and training. How you communicate your oral health message, deciding on the approach you wish to use for a particular patient will dictate your success. You will need to be knowledgeable about dental diseases, their cause and prevention. Your initial training will probably not be sufficient and you may need to study further.

The National Examining Board for Dental Nurses Qualification Certificate in Oral Health Education would be a good one to achieve.

TOP TIPS
1. Avoid using jargon when talking to patients.
2. Use only three to four key points when putting your message across.
3. Check that your message has been understood.

LINKS WITH OTHER CHAPTERS
- Chapter 15 – Medical Emergencies.
- Chapter 20 – Periodontal Treatment and Prevention of Dental Disease.

REFERENCES
Ireland, R. (ed.) (2004) *Advanced Dental Nursing*. Blackwell Publishing, Oxford (Chapter 2, Oral Health Education, and Chapter 3, Special Care Dentistry).
General Dental Council Guidance Booklets. (2006) *Principles of Complaint Handling*. General Dental Council, London. Available on the General Dental Council website (http://www.gdc-uk.org) under guidance documents.
General Dental Council Guidance Booklets. (2006) *Principles of Raising Concerns*. General Dental Council, London. Available on the General Dental Council website (http://www.gdc-uk.org) under guidance documents.
Lambden, P. (ed.) (2002) *Dental Law and Ethics*. Radcliffe Medical Press, Oxford.

Managing Dental Records

Whether you are working in a National Health Service (NHS) general dental practice, private practice, or community or hospital service it is essential to have a set of full patient records available for each visit.

WHY ARE DENTAL RECORDS IMPORTANT?

The patient's dental record should be:

- up to date;
- accurate;
- in a logical order;
- legible (in ink not in pencil).

The records are important because:

- Omissions or mistakes could lead to the patient receiving the wrong treatment or failing to receive necessary treatment.
- In the event of a medico-legal case, professional indemnity organisations have advised that the better the patient's dental records the easier it is to defend the case!
- Under NHS Regulations a dentist can be asked to produce a patient's records within 14 days, at the request of the Dental Practice Board (now Business Services Authority), a Health Authority or the Secretary of State for Health.
- Dental records may also be a valuable resource when establishing the identity of an accident victim or in a police enquiry.

WHAT INFORMATION IS NEEDED FOR A COMPLETE DENTAL RECORD?

A patient's record must contain accurate details of:

- the care and treatment given to each patient (under the NHS this could be a 'unit of dental activity');
- referrals;
- occasional/emergency treatment;
- radiographs;
- photographs;
- study models.

It is good practice to also include:

- form with personal details and contact information;
- copy of patient's treatment plan;
- copy of patient's agreement to private treatment;
- medical/dental history with doctor's contact;
- treatment undertaken by a dental hygienist/therapist or other dental care professional;
- requests and results of pathology tests etc.;
- payment details;
- attendance record – failed to attend/late;
- prescriptions given;
- laboratory work sent and received;
- general correspondence.

A–Z OF DENTAL RECORDS

Access to Information Act

This Act allows patients access to information held about them whether on paper or on computer. Access is usually granted on receipt of a written request.

Age of consent (see Consent)

The law defines the age of consent to be from the eighteenth birthday. Children between 16 and 17 years are entitled to give consent for surgical and medical procedures. Children under the age of 16 may be capable of giving informed consent, and their wishes must be respected above those of their parents. It is good practice to obtain consent of both child and parent. When an adult does not have the intellectual capacity to understand and consent then it is admissible for a carer or relative to be involved in the decision. The treatment must be in the best interest of the patient. In 1990 the Access to Medical Records Act gave patients the right to access their personal medical and dental records including radiographs. Further information can be found on the Department of Health's website (www.doh.gov.uk).

Alphabetical filing

This system of filing is usually used for storing patient record cards and means each individual record can be found using the patient's name.

Chronological filing

This method of filing is usually used for the recall system in some dental practices and is a method of storing recall cards in date order to facilitate the sending out of recall cards at the appropriate time.

Computer records

Many dental practices now maintain computerised clinical records, this system may be valuable in reducing the amount of paper and contribute to ease of access when locating patient information. It is essential to have a reliable back-up system. It is also important to check that the quality of radiographs and photographs are of a high standard and that dental and periodontal charts can be clearly reproduced to comply with NHS regulations and the General Dental Council's document *Maintaining Standards*.

Confidentiality

Information gained during the course of a patient's dental care and treatment is confidential. Information (even the date and time of a patient's appointment) should not be divulged to another person as a breach in confidentiality may lead to a case of professional misconduct being brought against you.

Consent

In legal terms every person of sound mind and body has the right to decide and consent to what is being done to his/her body. Treating a patient without their consent may be considered a civil or legal offence. Obtaining valid consent is not just a one-off conversation, it can be implied, expressed in writing or orally. The patient must be capable of making an informed choice about their treatment. Before a dental procedure is carried out the following points need to be discussed with the patient in terms that they understand:

- reason for the treatment being recommended;
- details of the procedure;
- benefits of the treatment;
- risks involved;
- possible discomfort;
- alternative treatment options;
- consequences of not having the treatment.

Patient consent must be documented in the patient's records by the dentist and for treatment under dental sedation, written consent should be obtained and a copy kept in the patient's records.

Data protection

Data protection legislation protects the individual from having their personal information circulated or made available to third parties without their consent. Precautions must be taken to ensure that personal information is not made available to anyone else, even accidentally.

Dental charting

Dental charting forms a crucial part of the patient's records. If you need a reminder of the Standard UK charting used to record restorations, extractions, crowns and root canal therapy, see Chapter 3. Incorrect or insufficient charting may lead to a hearing in front of the General Dental Council's Conduct Committee like this one reported in the *GDC Gazette*: 'a dentist who failed to supply a full dental charting and reporting on periodontal status on a DPB claim form and failings in practice administration'. The dentist was found guilty of serious professional misconduct.

FDI Charting (two-digit system)
This system was designed by the Federation Dentaire Internationale (FDI; International Dental Federation) to establish a standardised method which could be used worldwide (see Chapter 3).

Medical history
A full medical history should be taken by the clinician before starting a course of treatment and checked each time a new course of treatment occurs. A medical history checklist can be completed by the patient alone or by the patient with the help of a trained staff member. The completed checklist should always be checked and confirmed by the dentist.

If you notice any sign indicating a medical condition which would affect the patient's treatment, you should tell the dentist (see Chapter 3).

Periodontal charting
Periodontal charting is used to record the periodontal condition in terms of pocket depth and tooth mobility (see Chapter 3). Tooth mobility is recorded for each tooth on a scale of 0 to 3.

Radiographs
Any radiographs taken should be filed either in the patient's record card with their name and date marked on them or mounted in a separate file with sufficient patient details to allow them to be found when required (see Chapter 4).

Security
It is essential that patient records are kept secure whether currently in use or archived. Locked filing cabinets are an effective way of securing paper records and password protection will ensure that computer-held records are only available to the people who are entitled to view them.

Study models

Study models taken for the patient should be kept in a way that protects them from damage and marked in way that allows them to be easily found when required.

Medical Emergencies

15

> In the event of a patient becoming ill in the dental
> surgery, the dental nurse must be able to act
> quickly to help prevent the illness or injury from
> becoming worse.

When a patient enters the surgery the full responsibility for his/her health, safety and welfare is in the hands of the dentist and the team. A patient may become ill at any time while in the surgery, and this could be as a result of dental treatment or due to an existing illness.

It is most important that the dental nurse is able to recognise signs and symptoms, minimise the risk of an emergency and assist the dentist if an emergency arises.

WHY COULD AN EMERGENCY HAPPEN?
- Anxiety, stress, nervousness.
- Pain.
- Inadequate medical history obtained.
- Medical history not routinely updated.
- A reaction to local anaesthetic.
- Physical exertion.
- Patient did not understand or carry out post-operative instructions.
- Patient's existing medical condition.
- The result of an unplanned occurrence – accident.

WHAT EMERGENCIES ARE THE MOST COMMON?
- Fainting (syncope) is the most common.
- Fainting during sedation.
- Anaphylactic shock.

- Diabetic hypoglycaemia.
- Epileptic attack.
- Cardiac arrest.
- Stroke.
- Shock.
- Choking or difficulty breathing.
- Asthmatic attack.
- Haemorrhage.
- Burns/scalds.

MINIMISE THE RISK

Emergencies must be eliminated where possible, it is far better to avoid the occurrence than have to deal with them. The risk can be minimised in a variety of ways.

Reception
- Create a relaxed and pleasant atmosphere.
- Greet patient with a smile and be pleasant.
- Be aware of their apprehensions, make conversation to alleviate any fears.
- Give the patient your full attention.

Surgery
- Ensure surgery is well ventilated.
- Talk to the patient, give a brief explanation of the dental procedure.
- Ask patient to remove heavy outer clothing.
- Check and update medical history under the dentist's direct supervision.
- Ensure any pre-operative instructions have been followed.
- Allow the patient to stop and interrupt the procedure.
- Observe and reassure the patient throughout.
- Provide efficient chairside support, e.g. protect soft tissues, aspirate carefully.
- Be responsive to the dentist's and patient's needs.
- Observe the patient and inform the dentist if you recognise changes in condition.

- Ensure all post-operative instructions are given both verbally and in writing.
- Do not allow the patient to leave until they are fit to do so.

The whole dental team can be part of this procedure which starts when the patient enters the reception area and is greeted by the receptionist and terminating when they are dismissed from the practice on the instruction of the dentist.

EMERGENCY PROCEDURES

It is not always possible to eliminate an emergency even if you have carried out all procedures to minimise the risk. The dental team must be prepared to act if an emergency situation arises – a well-planned rehearsed routine saves lives.

Preparation

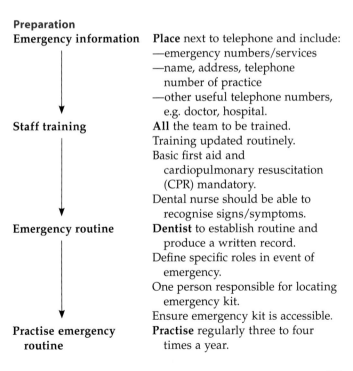

Emergency information **Place** next to telephone and include:
—emergency numbers/services
—name, address, telephone number of practice
—other useful telephone numbers, e.g. doctor, hospital.

Staff training **All** the team to be trained.
Training updated routinely.
Basic first aid and cardiopulmonary resuscitation (CPR) mandatory.
Dental nurse should be able to recognise signs/symptoms.

Emergency routine **Dentist** to establish routine and produce a written record.
Define specific roles in event of emergency.
One person responsible for locating emergency kit.
Ensure emergency kit is accessible.

Practise emergency routine **Practise** regularly three to four times a year.

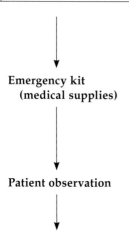

Ensure staff are aware of and
capable of specific roles.

Ensure staff competently work as
a team.

Emergency kit (medical supplies)

Store where readily available.

Appointed/trained person
responsible for kit.

Check supplies routinely, e.g.
expiry dates.

Maintain record of contents.

Drugs used replaced immediately.

Patient observation

Observe patient's condition
throughout treatment.

Be able to recognise vital signs, e.g.
pallor, breathing difficulties, pain.

COMMON EMERGENCIES

Fainting (syncope)

Causes: Reduced blood supply to the brain caused by: anxiety, pain, hunger, fatigue, and high temperature.

Signs/symptoms:

- pale/clammy skin;
- slow feeble pulse;
- shivering;
- sighing;
- loss of consciousness;
- hot;
- thirsty;
- black and white vision;
- dizziness.

Action:

(1) lower head, feet raised higher;
(2) loosen tight clothing;
(3) check pulse;

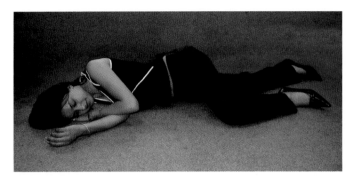

Fig. 15.1 Recovery position.

(4) if necessary place in recovery position when casualty regains consciousness (Figure 15.1);

(5) record all details on patient's medical history form.

15

Fainting during sedation
Causes: analgesic overdose; deficiency of oxygen; respiratory failure.

Signs/symptoms:

- pale, clammy skin;
- feeble pulse.

Action:

(1) sedation is stopped immediately;
(2) remove any obstructions from the mouth, clear airway;
(3) administer oxygen.

Anaphylactic shock
Cause: severe allergic reaction to a drug or agent.

Signs/symptoms:

- generalised itching, tingling;
- breathing difficulties;
- pale, cold, clammy skin;
- weak/rapid pulse;
- convulsions.

Action:

(1) lay patient flat;
(2) dentist administers intramuscular adrenaline, intravenous hydrocortisone, intramuscular chlorphenamine, oxygen;
(3) call ambulance;
(4) observe patient's airway as fluid can collect in the larynx causing swelling;
(5) if the patient's condition deteriorates and there is complete loss of blood pressure and/or no pulse present administer CPR.

Diabetic hypoglycaemia

Cause: blood sugar level falls below normal.
   Signs/symptoms:

- sudden onset;
- profuse sweating;
- aggressive/excitable/irritable/restless;
- rapid feeble pulse;
- headache;
- sweet smell on breath;
- palpitations.

Action:

(1) lay patient flat;
(2) administer sugar orally;
(3) if patient loses consciousness dentist administers intravenous glucose.

Epileptic attack

Causes: various: hereditary, accident, injury during birth, severe infection, high fever causing damage.
   Signs/symptoms:

- Initial stage: **aura phase** – irritable, headache.
- Second stage: **tonic phase** – spasms, loss of consciousness.
- Third stage: **clonic phase** – uncontrolled jerking, convulsions.

Action:

(1) protect patient from hurting themselves;
(2) move all equipment out of the way;
(3) protect patient's head;
(4) observe breathing and check pulse;
(5) if fit does not stop after few minutes dentist administers intravenous diazepam and oxygen;
(6) call ambulance.

Cardiac arrest
Cause: severe hypotension; myocardial infarction; oxygen deficiency.

Signs/symptoms:

- pale/clammy skin, grey complexion;
- pulse is absent and breathlessness;
- loss of consciousness;
- severe crushing pain across chest, radiating into the left arm.

Action:

(1) summon ambulance immediately;
(2) support patient's back and head with pillows;
(3) dentist administers oxygen and nitrous oxide;
(4) have suction ready in case of vomiting;
(5) be prepared to administer CPR if trained to required level (Figures 15.2 and 15.3).

Stroke
Causes: sudden interruption to the blood supply to the brain; ruptured blood vessels; thrombosis; hypertension.

Signs/symptoms:

- loss of consciousness;
- weakness of arm and or leg on one side causing partial paralysis;
- partial paralysis on one side of face causing it to droop.

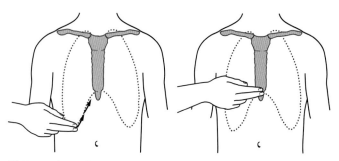

(1) Trace along rib cage to notch
(2) Place middle finger on notch and index finger beside it

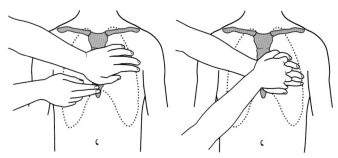

(3) Measure by placing one hand beside the index finger of the other hand
(4) Link fingers and keep them up off the chest

Fig. 15.2 Cardiopulmonary resuscitation (CPR) hand positions.

Action:

(1) call ambulance immediately;
(2) keep airway clear;
(3) keep patient in horizontal position, head raised, support body;
(4) dentist administers oxygen.

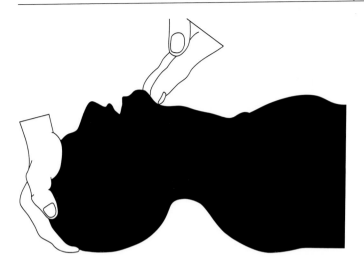

Push back on the forehead and use the other hand to lift the chin

Fig. 15.3 Head tilt.

Shock

Causes: loss of body fluids, e.g. haemorrhage, hypotension; bacterial infection in the bloodstream; anaphylaxis; emotional shock.

Signs/symptoms:

- similar to those of fainting, plus the following:
- dry mouth;
- dilated pupils;
- reduced flow of urine.

Action:

(1) call ambulance immediately;
(2) keep patient warm.

Choking/difficulty breathing

Causes: obstruction by an inhaled object, e.g. endodontic instrument, fragment of tooth or filling material.

Sign/symptoms:

- difficulty breathing;
- patient is choking.

Action:

(1) encourage patient to cough;
(2) try to remove with the aspirator;
(3) give several sharp blows between the shoulder blades;
(4) if all the above fails dentist performs the Heimlich manoeuvre by standing behind the casualty and placing hands between the navel and rib cage and giving a sudden thrust (Figure 15.4);
(5) refer patient to hospital for chest X-ray.

Asthmatic attack

Causes: anxiety; infection; allergic reaction.

Signs/symptoms:

- wheezing;
- difficulty breathing;
- tightness in the chest;
- patient may appear anxious.

Action:

(1) instruct patient to use their own medication, e.g. salbutamol inhaler;
(2) calm the patient, encourage them to relax;
(3) in severe cases dentist administers intravenous hydrocortisone and oxygen;
(4) call ambulance.

Haemorrhage

(For further information on the stages of haemorrhage see Chapter 7.)

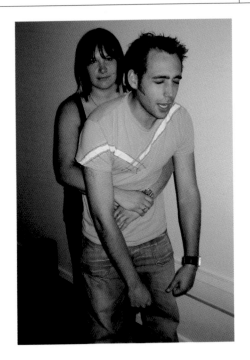

Fig. 15.4 Heimlich manoeuvre.

Cause: usually associated with extraction of a tooth.

Signs/symptoms:

- profuse bleeding from the operation site;
- bleeding continues to occur for a long period of time.

Action:

(1) place sterile pressure pad over the operation site and ask patient to bite firmly;
(2) if bleeding persists suturing may be required to hold the tissues together.

Burns/scalds

Causes: direct contact with the flame from a Bunsen burner; handling a hot dry instrument; spillage of a chemical substance onto the skin or steam from the autoclave.

Signs/symptoms:

- redness, swelling and blistering of the skin;
- may be painful;
- if peeling or charred and skin looks grey, but not painful it may be deep and serious.*

Action:

(1) if possible remove any constricting items, e.g. rings, watches or clothing before swelling occurs;
(2) cool the area under slow running water for 10 minutes or longer if pain continues;
(3) cover the burn with sterile dressing.

If signs/symptoms present as above (*), cover burn and refer to hospital.

TOP TIPS

1. Ensure patient's medical history is reviewed at each and every appointment, e.g. ask the patient if there have been any changes since the last time they attended.
2. Remember the dentist is in charge of all emergency situations, the dental nurse is required to assist under the direction of the dentist.
3. Do not attempt to administer first aid or emergency aid unless you have been trained to do so.
4. The purpose of emergency aid is to: preserve life; prevent the condition worsening; promote recovery.
5. Practise emergency procedures regularly.
6. Ensure you receive adequate and appropriate training frequently so that you can provide competent assistance in the event of an emergency.

7. All emergencies and accidents must be entered into the accident book and records held in accordance with the Data Protection Act.

LINKS TO OTHER CHAPTERS
- Chapter 16 – Health and Safety in the Dental Environment.
- Chapter 6 – Extractions.
- Chapter 7 – Minor Oral Surgery.

15

Health and Safety in the Dental Environment

Health and safety is concerned with protecting people while they are at work. This is achieved by taking the correct precautions to prevent employees, self-employed visitors and members of the public from being harmed or becoming ill.

MANAGEMENT OF HEALTH AND SAFETY
Your employer is legally required to manage health and safety. This is carried out by adopting five key steps (Figure 16.1):

(1) Devise a health and safety policy
(2) Organise the team
(3) Set health and safety standards and implement safety systems
(4) Monitor health and safety performance
(5) Implement Review and Audit systems and revise if necessary

STEP 1 – HEALTH AND SAFETY POLICY
- All dental establishments regardless of the size or number of people employed must have a policy for managing health and safety.
- Where five or more people are employed at any one time, the policy must be in writing.
- The policy must be brought to the attention of all employees and reviewed and revised as and when necessary.
- A clearly defined policy that is used in the day-to-day operations of the organisation assists employers in complying with legislation and maintaining workplace standards.

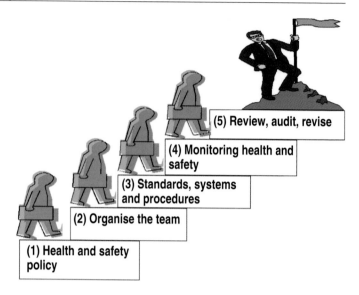

Fig. 16.1 Five steps to health and safety management.

- Employers are required to consult with the team prior to implementing or revising a policy. This provides the opportunity for people to discuss, seek advice and take an active part in ensuring the policy is workable.
- The policy generally consists of three parts:
  −a statement of commitment;
  −details of individual responsibilities;
  −details of the arrangements for health and safety.

Part 1 – statement of commitment

This is the section that specifies the organisation's intention to ensure the health, safety and welfare of employees (both direct and self-employed) and anyone else who may be affected by its activities. The most senior person must sign it. In a general dental practice this will normally be the employer, however, in larger organisations it may be a managing director.

Part 2 – responsibilities

Everyone has a responsibility for ensuring health and safety at work, but the overall and final responsibility for the action of employees is that of the employer. On a daily basis the actual responsibility for ensuring that the policy in place is put into practice is often delegated to a 'suitable and appropriate' person, e.g. a practice manager. Other people may also have day-to-day responsibilities for specific duties, e.g. a dental nurse may be responsible for monitoring the control of waste or a dental receptionist for monitoring the incidence of violence and aggression from patients.

Part 3 – arrangements

This section of the policy covers specific hazards within the workplace and the established precautions in place aimed at controlling risks arising from hazards. Employers are legally required to carry out risk assessments, and where there are five or more employees the assessment must be recorded. Risk assessments should be incorporated into the health and safety policy by addressing them as individual arrangements. The following list includes 'generic' arrangements, which are relevant to all dental environments, however, each policy should reflect an individual organisation.

ARRANGEMENTS FOR HEALTH AND SAFETY

Accident and first aid

- All accidents, including near-misses and work-related illnesses, should be reported to a named person.
- An investigation should be undertaken to determine the underlying cause/s and determine the most appropriate controls to prevent recurrence.
- An accident record should be completed which includes specific details, this must be kept confidential under the Data Protection Act which restricts access to the information (Figure 16.2).
- The accident may need to be reported to the enforcing authority under RIDDOR (Reporting of Injuries Diseases Dangerous

ACCIDENT REPORT FORM

(A) The accident report form contains personal details that must be kept confidential in compliance with the Data Protection Act. After completion, **Part B** must be passed to the person responsible for record storage and kept for a period of at least three years from the date the accident happened.

Name of Person who had the accident:...

Accident No:..

✂..

(B) 1. Who is completing this form? (please circle) (A) Person who had the accident

(B) Someone else (please record details below)

Name:..

Address:..

Tel no: ....

Relationship/Association to the person who had the accident...

2. Person who had the accident (please circle) Employee/Self-employed   Visitor   Patient   Other

(please specify)..

Name:..

Home address:..

Tel no:...

Occupation:...

3. When did the accident happen: dd/mm/yy...

4. Where did the accident happen (exact location):...

5. What circumstances led to the accident happening?...

....

6. What were the consequences of the accident, e.g. injury, disease, ill-health, time lost by casualty?

....

7. Was any first aid treatment administered? (please circle)   YES (If yes please complete sections below) NO

Treatment administered:...

Who administered treatment and their position:..

8. What happened to the casualty following the accident, e.g. sent home, referred to hospital, etc?

....

9. The person completing this accident report form and the casualty (if these are different) must sign and date in the spaces provided.

The information contained in this document is a true and accurate account of the accident.

(A) SIGNATURE: Person completing the accident record form:...

(B) SIGNATURE: Person who had the accident:..

10. Is this accident reportable under RIDDOR? (please circle) YES NO

Date reported to the enforcing authority..

Name and position of person reporting to enforcing authority..

Fig. 16.2 Accident report form.

Occurrence Regulations 1995). These are accidents that result in:

–death;

–major injuries, dangerous occurrences or a work related disease as specified;

–an injury which results in an employee being off work for more than three days;

–an accident that results in a member of the public needing to visit hospital.

- The organisation should have as a minimum requirement recommended under the First Aid at Work Regulations, a first-aid box and an appointed person to ensure a casualty receives prompt medical attention. (See Further reading – RIDDOR explained.)
- **Minimum** contents of a first-aid box:

–general guidance leaflet;

–individually wrapped sterile adhesive dressings;

–sterile eye pads;

–individually wrapped sterile triangular bandages;

–safety pins;

–medium- and large-sized individually wrapped sterile unmedicated wound dressings;

–one pair of disposable gloves.

Emergency procedures, fire and evacuation

- A risk assessment will identify how the emergency may happen, how it can be prevented or the risks are minimised, e.g. a fire may start when flammable substances are stored on top of a central heating boiler causing the substance to ignite, the oxygen from the atmosphere will then cause the fire to spread.
- There should be a means of detecting any emergency, including fire. If a fire is detected, raising the alarm will be the first course of action.
- Action on discovering a fire and action on hearing the alarm should be displayed and communicated (Figure 16.3).
- Appropriate fire fighting equipment must be in place and regularly maintained (Figure 16.4).

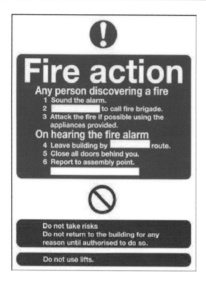

Fig. 16.3 Fire action sign.

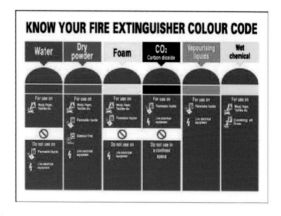

Fig. 16.4 Fire extinguishers.

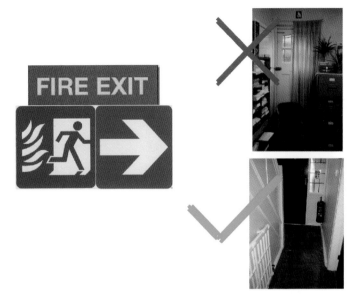

Fig. 16.5 Evacuation sign exit routes must be kept clear.

16

- Evacuation signs must be displayed and exit routes kept clear (Figure 16.5).
- Evacuation procedures should be practised regularly, a record kept and a named person responsible for co-ordinating the activity.

Hazardous substances

- All hazardous substances must be identified to determine if there is any risk of harm during day-to-day work activities. Control of Substances Hazardous to Health Regulations (COSHH) requires risk assessments to be carried out in certain circumstances.
- These might include manufactured chemicals which are labelled as hazardous, e.g. mercury, or substances as a result of the work being carried out, e.g. biological substances such as bacteria or viruses (Figure 16.6).

(a)   (b)

Fig. 16.6 (a) Hazardous substance and (b) hazard warning signs.

- Once a substance has been identified, a thorough assessment should be undertaken to determine who may be exposed and how the substance could cause harm – this could be through inhalation, absorption through skin, ingestion or splashing into the eyes.
- The assessment should examine the use, handling, storage, disposal and transportation of all hazardous substances. This will help to determine how substances should be controlled to reduce the risk of injury and ill-health.
- Biological substances may be assessed as part of the practice 'Infection Control Policy' which should include the following items:
  – immunisation;
  – personal protective equipment/clothing includes anything worn or held by a person;
  – single-use items;
  – decontamination, storage of dental equipment/instruments;
  – waste disposal;
  – laboratory procedures;

−safe working practices;
−medical history;
−spillages and inoculation injuries;
−personal hygiene;
−staff training.

Work equipment

- A range of equipment exists in dental environments including: chairs, reception desks, paper shredders, autoclaves, compressors, light cures and hand instruments to mention just a few.
- Generic safety procedures apply to all equipment regardless of its purpose, the way it is used and by whom, these include:
  −select and provide the correct equipment for the specific purpose;
  −determine safe working procedures and communicate to users;
  −have a pro-active system of maintenance, inspection and testing;
  −provide information, instruction and training which is periodically reviewed;
  −specific requirements apply for pressure vessels, e.g. autoclaves and compressor.

Ionising radiation

This is used in dentistry to take X-rays and provided it is controlled as specified in the Regulations it should not pose a risk. The Regulations require employers to take the following precautions:

- Appointment of a radiation protection advisor (RPA) and a radiation protection supervisor (RPS).
- Notification to the Health and Safety Executive of the equipment in use.
- Maintenance of equipment and record keeping.
- Justification for taking X-rays.
- Implementation of a quality assurance programme.

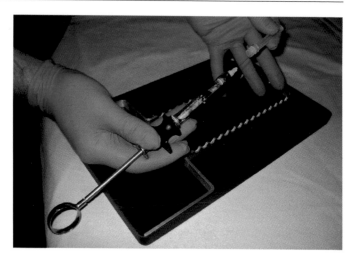

Fig. 16.7 Hazard resheathing local anaesthetic syringe.

- Provision of local rules.
- Prohibitions and restrictions.
- Information, instruction and training for all staff working with ionising radiation.

RISK ASSESSMENT

A risk assessment is a means of examining what in your workplace could cause harm to people, to help you decide if you have taken sufficient precautions or you need to do more in order to prevent accidents.

The process of carrying out a risk assessment is relatively straightforward and involves the following stages:

(1) Identify hazards – a hazard is something, which has the potential to cause harm, e.g. re-sheathing a local anaesthetic syringe (Figure 16.7).
(2) Assess the risks – risk is the likelihood that the hazard will cause harm. This will depend upon a number of factors including: who is exposed to the hazard and how many

people, how often are they exposed, how might the hazard cause harm and what are the consequences, what existing precautions/controls are in place and are these adequate and suitable?

(3) Introduce further controls – where the hazard cannot be removed control measures must be introduced to reduce the risk of the accident happening and limit the consequences, e.g. the use of needle guards or a device which removes the needle from the syringe. Both methods isolate the person from the hazard (Figure 16.8a, b).

(4) Record the findings – as previously mentioned where five or more people are employed it is a legal requirement to record the findings, however, even if there are fewer than five it is helpful to keep a record.

(5) Review and revise – risk assessments should be reviewed periodically to help determine if the controls are still working, if not why not and what else needs to be done.

The legal requirement for risk assessments includes assessing risks for new and expectant mothers and young persons (those under 18 years).

16

Working environment

Regardless of where you work and the type of workplace, generic issues need to be considered in order to ensure the health, safety and welfare of employees and others who may enter the premises. Consideration should be given to the following:

• Design and structure of premises taking into consideration the type of work activities being undertaken and the layout and space inside the building.
• Stair and floor surfaces to ensure safe movement within the building avoiding the risk of slips, trips and falls.
• Doors and windows which can be cleaned safely and opened without endangering people.
• Ventilation, heating and lighting should be appropriate for the type of work being undertaken.
• Workstations and seating must be suitable for the individual task and people using them.

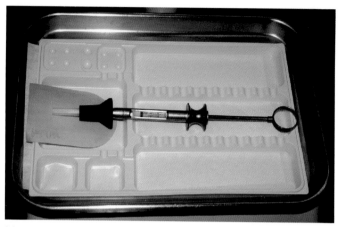

(a)

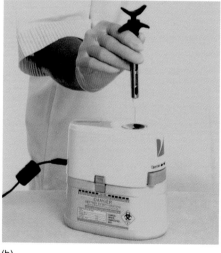

(b)

Fig. 16.8 (a,b) Risk control – isolating the risk. (Reproduced with permission from CooleyField & Associates Ltd.)

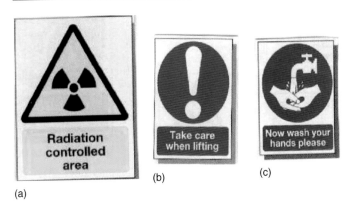

(a)

(b)

(c)

Fig. 16.9 Safety signs. (a) Warning sign. (b,c) Mandatory signs.

- Maintenance and housekeeping to ensure premises remain structurally sound and kept clean and tidy.
- Safety signs should be displayed where necessary to communicate information, e.g. a triangular sign depicting a black pictogram on an yellow background is to warn people of a hazard such as an ionising radiation sign, and a round sign depicting a white pictogram on a blue background informs people of something that is mandatory (Figure 16.9).
- Welfare facilities must be provided to include: toilets, washing and drying facilities, drinking water, clothing storage, changing facilities and staff rest areas.
- Safe storage and stacking facilities to reduce the risk of items being stacked too high or in unsafe places.

Manual handling

All dental environments need to carry out some form of manual handling involving the movement of objects, e.g. stock, equipment or people. If possible, the movement of any loads should be avoided. However, if this is unavoidable and the risk of injury is likely, then a risk assessment approach must be taken using the following process.

- Load – analyse the load including weight, shape, height, stability and determine how the risk of injury can be prevented or reduced.
- Individual capabilities – has the person/s carrying out the task received training, do they have the necessary capabilities and are there any health or medical conditions that may put them more at risk?
- Task – what is involved in the movement of the load. Does it involve twisting, stooping, lifting, carrying distances, repetitive movements or is force required? Determine how the task can be designed to prevent injury.
- Environment – look at where the task is taking place, is there sufficient space, is the flooring suitable, are there any obstructions and is the lighting sufficient?

If it is not possible to avoid manual handling tasks then correct handling techniques must be followed (Figure 16.10):

- Plan and prepare the activity, consider what is being moved, check the weight of the load.
- Position yourself with feet slightly apart distributing your weight evenly.
- Lift by bending the knees, keeping the back straight, get a firm grip around the base of the load and lift in stages.
- Move the load keeping it close to the body and ensure you can see where you are going.
- Lower the load by reversing the lift movement, avoid putting the load down on fingers or toes and ensure it is secure in its final position.

Waste disposal
- Dental establishments produce three main types of waste:
  - Hazardous or clinical, e.g. contaminated with body fluids from a known infectious patient, amalgam waste, radiographic solutions, etc. Put in yellow approved sacks/rigid containers.
  - Non-hazardous, e.g. waste produced during treatment of a non-infectious patient etc. Put in yellow or yellow/black sacks (Tiger sacks).

–Domestic waste, e.g. paper, packaging, etc. Put in black sacks.

- Assessments must be undertaken to determine the quantity and type of waste being produced and removed from premises.
- Premises producing hazardous or clinical waste must notify the Environment Agency.

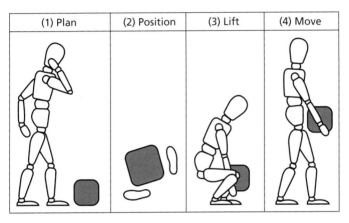

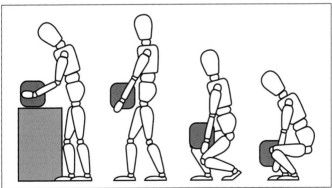

Fig. 16.10 Correct handling techniques.

- Waste must be segregated as listed above, stored and disposed of correctly and safely.
- It is illegal to mix hazardous waste with non-hazardous waste.
- Records and consignment notes must be held of waste disposal and transfer.

(At the time of writing hazardous waste is under consultation with the Department of Health, therefore, changes may come into force.)

Display screen equipment
- The use of computers in dental establishments has increased over the past five years. Employers are required to ensure they are used safely without risk to a person's health.
- Employers are required to identify which people are using computers and analyse the work being carried out.
- An assessment should be made to include the workstation, work equipment, work activities, environmental issues, i.e. lighting and layout.
- The assessment will identify if changes are required.
- Employees must be trained on the safe use of computers and what to do if they experience any problems.
- The employer may have to provide eye sight tests on the request of the display screen equipment user.

Everyone in the workplace plays an important part in managing health and safety on a daily basis in order to ensure the policy works.

In this section we have dealt with some, but not all, of the more common issues that relate to all dental environments. By following the guidance given and taking practical steps, accidents can be prevented.

STEP 2 – ORGANISE THE TEAM
- Your employer will have overall **control** of all health and safety aspects associated with the day-to-day operation of the organisation.

- Every member of staff has a responsibility for ensuring their own health and safety and has a duty of care to others. All staff must **co-operate** with each other to ensure health and safety is a team approach.
- Your employer must ensure you are **competent** to carry out your role safely. This could mean that you need specific training on a range of tasks. Those who have delegated responsibilities for health and safety, i.e. first aiders, must have the knowledge and skills to carry out this role.
- There must be a system of **communicating** health and safety, this could be at team meetings or focus groups. Staff should be able to consult through all levels of the organisation on aspects that affect them. Means of consultation should be clearly set out.

STEP 3 – SET STANDARDS AND IMPLEMENT SAFE SYSTEMS

- Acceptable standards of health and safety must be clearly defined and state how the standards are going to be achieved.
- The policy should describe in detail who does what and how, this is more commonly known as 'safe working procedures'.
- Risk assessments will highlight where improvements need to be made, how they will be implemented and when.
- All members of the team should be involved in identifying hazards and how to control the risk of injury or harm.

STEP 4 – MONITORING HEALTH AND SAFETY PERFORMANCE

There are several ways to monitor how you are meeting the standards set and to measure your performance in terms of health and safety:

- Workplace inspections are a useful 'tool' for highlighting issues. Areas can be inspected using a simple checklist and the results acted on accordingly.
- The frequency that the engineers are called out can be collated.
- Accident figures should be analysed.
- Information from practice meetings and focus groups will help determine how well the practice is performing.

From the information gathered, decide if there are any differences in what is actually happening and the standards that are set.

STEP 5 – REVIEW, AUDIT AND REVISE SYSTEMS
- Health and safety management will only work in practice if it is continuously reviewed.
- The previous four steps need to be audited regularly and revised if necessary.
- Revision may be required if significant changes have happened in the organisation, i.e. a new piece of equipment, change to working practices as determined by the profession or a new member of staff has joined the team.
- All staff should be involved in agreeing changes to ensure they are realistic, practical and achievable.

SUMMARY
Dental nurses have both legal and ethical obligations to take part in the management of health and safety in the workplace. Statutory registration places responsibilities on you for the protection of patients, both in the treatment provided and their health, safety and welfare while they are in the practice.

You may want to use the checklist at the end of this chapter to 'test' how well your practice is managing health and safety to determine if there are any areas that need clarification (Figure 16.11).

Dental nurses must ensure they are carrying out their legal and ethical duties and avoid actions that could put themselves or others at risk of injury, ill-health or potential litigious situations.

> **TOP TIPS**
> 1. Obtain a copy of your health and safety policy, or ensure you have immediate access to the document.
> 2. Find out what each team member is responsible for.

Use the checklist to 'test' how well your practice is managing health and safety and determine if there are any areas that you need to address with the practice manager/principal.

QUESTION	YES	NO	ACTION
(1) Health and safety policy			
(a) Do we have a written health and safety policy?			
(b) Have you been informed of the contents of the policy?			
(c) Is the policy up to date?			
(d) Does the policy contain a statement of commitment?			
(e) Does the policy clearly show who is responsible for what?			
(f) Does the policy set out how we arrange for health and safety?			
(g) Is the policy suitable and sufficient for our requirements?			
(2) Organise the team			
(a) Do we have a system for communicating health and safety?			
(b) Has your competence been assessed and your training needs identified?			
(c) Does someone take control of health and safety issues?			
(d) Do you work together as a team to ensure health and safety?			
(3) Standards, systems and procedures			
(a) Have risk assessments been conducted?			
(b) Are the results of risk assessment communicated to you?			
(c) Have we got safe operating procedures for 'at risk tasks'?			
(d) Are risks adequately controlled throughout the practice?			
(e) Are we actively involved in making the practice safer?			

Fig. 16.11 Managing health and safety checklist. (*Continued overleaf*)

QUESTION	YES	NO	ACTION
(4) Monitoring health and safety performance			
(a) Do we carry out health and safety inspections internally?			
(b) Do we act on the results of the inspections?			
(c) Do we report and record all cases of accidents?			
(d) Do we investigate all accidents including near-misses?			
(e) Do we take action to prevent further accidents occurring?			
(f) Do we discuss health and safety at team meetings?			
(g) Do we know how often we have equipment failures?			
(h) Are we monitoring our health and safety performance?			
(5) Review, audit and revise systems			
(a) Do we have a procedure for reviewing health and safety?			
(b) Do we discuss the need for improvements?			
(c) Do we revise systems and procedure when necessary?			
(d) Do we agree any changes before they are actioned?			
(e) Are all members of the team involved in the formal review?			
General – safe and healthy environment			
(a) Do we work in premises that are safe?			
(b) Do we have adequate facilities to work safely?			
(c) Do we have an accident reporting procedure that works?			
(d) Do we have procedures for the safe use of equipment?			
(e) Do we have procedures for the safe use of substances?			
(f) Do we have general fire procedures?			
(g) Do we effectively manage health and safety?			

Fig. 16.11 *Continued*

3. Decide if you are complying with the arrangements for health and safety as set out in the policy, are you meeting the required standard?
4. Determine if your policy works for you and the team, does it reflect a true picture of what is happening?
5. Talk to your employer if you think the policy needs changing, discuss changes with the team and set objectives that can be measured within a set time period.
6. Include health and safety on the agenda at every practice meeting.
7. Take it in turns to research and discuss a specific topic relevant to health and safety.
8. Include health and safety training as part of your continuing professional development (CPD).

LINKS TO OTHER CHAPTERS
- Chapter 1 – Daily Routine Maintenance.
- Chapter 2 – Infection Control.
- Chapter 4 – Dental Radiography.

FURTHER READING

s4dental Cross Infection Control Dental Team Training. Schulke & Mayr UK Ltd.

Health and Safety Executive (2000) Ionising Radiation Regulations 1999, no. L121. ISBN 0717617467. ACOP*

Health and Safety Executive (2000) Management of Health and Safety at Work Regulations 1999, no. L21. ISBN 0717624889. ACOP*

Health and Safety Executive (2000) Pressure Safety Systems Regulations, no. L122. ISBN 071761767X.

Health and Safety Executive (1999) RIDDOR Explained, no. HSE 31. ISBN 0717624412.

*Approved Code of Practice – Approved by the Health and Safety Commission. ACOPs give practical advice on how to comply with the law.

Dental Nurse Qualifications

NATIONAL VOCATIONAL QUALIFICATIONS (NVQS) IN ORAL HEALTH CARE

Vocational qualifications are those that reflect the skills, knowledge and understanding an individual possesses in relation to a specific area of work. In order to be able to assess these fairly across all assessment and training centres and for each individual candidate, there are specific criteria attached to each. These criteria are called Occupational Standards. The Occupational Standards cover all the major aspects of an occupation including current best practice, the ability to adapt to future requirements, and the knowledge and understanding, which underpins competent performance.

In November 2000, Healthwork UK, the National Training Organisation for the health care sector, launched the National Occupational Standards for Oral Health Care. These Occupational Standards were developed by Healthwork UK (now Skills for Health) under direction from a steering group chaired by the General Dental Council, including representatives from the British Dental Association, British Association of Dental Nurses, National Examining Board for Dental Nurses (NEBDN) and Department of Health. They have been used to develop two National Vocational Qualifications for Oral Health Care; Level 2 – Support and Level 3 – Dental Nursing.

In 2006, the Occupational Standards are due to be reviewed in a project led by Skills for Health. It is likely that as a result of this project there will no longer be a Level 2 qualification and that the Level 3 will be restructured to meet the requirements of the General Dental Council's curriculum.

The qualifications currently can be tailored to the individual's working environment and include additional units for progression. They also include units from other sectors, which can then be used as accredited prior learning should the candidate choose to change careers.

The NEBDN jointly with City and Guilds Affinity and Scottish Qualifications Authority awards the oral health care qualifications. These organisations are jointly responsible for monitoring the assessment process and to undertake external verification of awards.

Centres wishing to provide these qualifications must first be accredited by City and Guilds. The accreditation process involves completing a self-assessment document about the centre's ability to provide the qualification and the suitability of the systems in place to fulfil this. On submission of the self-assessment documentation an external verifier arranges an appointment to verify the statements made in the self-assessment document and to monitor the availability and appropriateness of resources, systems, policies etc. Once accredited, assessment centres are given a centre number.

Students can access these NVQs by registering with an Accredited Assessment Centre. Once registered, the training and assessment of the student may be carried out in a variety of ways by different groups of people and the arrangements may vary from region to region or even from assessment centre to assessment centre. It is advisable to check these arrangements with your local assessment centre.

In order to gain an NVQ the student must continually demonstrate their ability to perform tasks, their understanding of the processes and associated theory and their ability to organise appropriate evidence into a portfolio. The student must also at some stage during their training have sat and passed the Independent Assessment – a written paper set and marked by the NEBDN.

To achieve the current NVQ Level 2 the candidate must compile a portfolio of evidence that demonstrates their ability and understanding across nine units (modules). Six of these units are mandatory and will be completed by every student undertaking the Level 2 and three are selected from the remaining five optional units. They must also complete a one-hour written paper which assesses their understanding of three of the six mandatory units.

To achieve the current Level 3 the candidate must compile a portfolio of evidence that demonstrates their ability and understanding across 14 units. Nine of these units are mandatory and will be completed by every student undertaking the Level 3, and five are selected from the remaining 24. They must also complete a two-hour written paper which assesses their understanding of six of the nine mandatory units.

A candidate's competence is assessed by one or more assessors who are occupationally competent, understand the occupational standards and hold the relevant assessor qualification. Quality of the qualifications is assured by (a) the Independent Assessment – no candidate can qualify on the say of the assessment centre alone and (b) the verification processes. Each Accredited Centre should have one person (internal verifier or internal verifier co-ordinator) who is responsible for monitoring the quality of each portfolio submitted, this is carried out using a thorough sampling system and ensuring the evidence clearly demonstrates validity, sufficiency, reliability, and authenticity. The internal verifier should also be occupationally competent, understand the occupational standards and hold the relevant verification qualification. The portfolios are then further checked by an external verifier who is an employee of City and Guilds and again uses sampling to monitor the decisions made by the internal verifier.

The two Oral Health Care NVQs do not have to be achieved progressively. A candidate does not have to do Level 2 before doing Level 3, although if they choose to do so some of the units are transferable and will not have to be repeated.

NATIONAL EXAMINING BOARD FOR DENTAL NURSES CERTIFICATE IN DENTAL NURSING

The British Dental Nurses and Assistants Examining Board was founded in 1943, but it was in 1936 that Mr Philip Grundy, a general practitioner from Leyland in Lancashire, first envisaged a qualifying examination for dental surgery assistants. The first examination was held in 1943 and has been held each year since, with the exception of the years 1947 and 1948. Since its inception in 1943 the NEBDN has become the most widely recognised awarding body for dental nurses in the UK.

Examiners for the Dental Nurse Certificate are selected from a panel of examiners. The panel of examiners is made up of registered dental nurses and dentists who have been qualified for more than seven years and demonstrate an active involvement in and commitment to the training and qualification of dental nurses. On appointment examiners are required to undergo a residential induction and training programme before examining.

The National Certificate is the standard achieved by the majority of dental nurses who qualify in this country. NEBDN continually monitors and reviews the structure of the qualification to ensure that it meets current educational requirements and the needs of the profession. To ensure that each candidate is given every opportunity to pass, candidates are assessed on each part of the examination by at least two members of the panel of examiners and the results of each individual examination centre moderated by a Presiding Examiner. The results from all the centres are then verified by the National Examination Committee.

The National Certificate Examination consists of five sections:

- written paper – part A;
- written paper – part B;
- spotter tests;
- practical;
- oral.

Each question in the examination is based on the syllabus available from the NEBDN (see Chapter 18 for contact details). The syllabus has 13 sections as detailed below.

(1) Health and Safety in the Workplace
(2) Emergencies in the Dental Surgery
(3) Legal and Ethical Issues in the Provision of Dental Care
(4) Anatomical Structures and Systems Relative to Dental Treatment

(5) Oral Disease and Pathology
(6) Patient Care and Management
(7) Assessing Patients' Oral Health Needs and Treating Planning
(8) Oral Health Promotion and Preventive Dentistry
(9) Restorative Dentistry
(10) Oral Surgery
(11) Orthodontic Procedures
(12) Dental Drugs, Materials, Instruments and Equipment
(13) Anaesthesia and Sedation in Relation to Dental Procedures

The syllabus details those areas of knowledge and understanding which a dental nurse needs to develop in order to be able to practise competently. Therefore much of the examination is based on the candidate being able to apply the knowledge in a practical setting.

The provision of dental nurse training is monitored for effectiveness by the Quality Assurance Service. The Quality Assurance Service is an integral part of the NEBDN and is responsible for the Quality Assurance and Accreditation of centres delivering training leading to all NEBDN qualifications.

It is important that any Awarding Body checks the suitability and capability of training providers to ensure that students are given the best possible opportunity to gain the qualification. The Standards required for accreditation have been divided into 32 criteria and a copy of the full standards and examples of evidence required can be obtained from the Quality Assurance Service Administrator.

REFERENCE
NEBDN website (www.nebdn.org.uk).

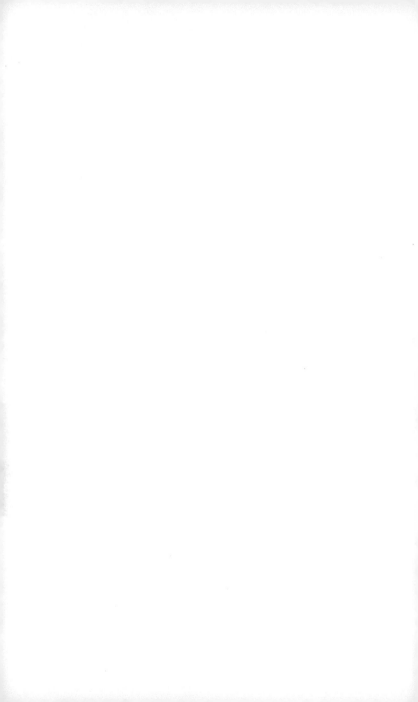

How to Improve Your Working Life

INTRODUCTION

This part of the handbook is devoted to you – the registered dental nurse or dental nurse in training. You probably didn't enter the profession for the money, the chances are you find the work interesting and varied, never boring, sometimes stressful and the patients and staff great!

During the past few years the status of the dental nursing profession and the potential for dental nurses to progress has been enhanced enormously. In this chapter the focus will be on you:

- Ensuring that you have the information you need to understand and benefit from the recent changes within dentistry; providing you with an update of the scope of practice of other dental care professionals (DCPs) in the dental team and your role within the team.
- Raising awareness of career options helping you make decisions about your future professional development.
- Providing a list of useful contacts and websites to support you in the future.

STATUTORY REGISTRATION – THE CHANGING DENTAL SCENE

Statutory Registration is not just a matter of gaining a qualification and signing the registration forms. Registration recognises the professional contribution made by dental nurses within the team. What does being a professional mean? A professional is a person doing something with great skill worthy of the high standards of a profession. A successful professional benefits others, has a fair degree of independence and is respected by his or her professional colleagues. Although Statutory Registration will bring strict regulation it will also provide a baseline of experienced competent staff, a building block which will allow us to:

- develop new roles and matching qualifications;
- expand our duties and merge roles;
- have the opportunity to influence future developments and play a more integrated role in the work of the General Dental Council (GDC) as a governing body.

Previously the Dentists Act had been rigorous in restricting the 'Practice of Dentistry' solely to dentists (with a few tasks delegated to dental hygienists and therapists). Now the new legislation has introduced a system in which all members of the clinical team have roles and responsibilities and are accountable for their own practice.

In future individuals and teams will be able to determine how duties can be undertaken using the wide range of competencies available in the Developing the Dental Team modular framework. In the future, DCPs will be able to practise dentistry within the limits of their competence.

How will registration affect you?

After the transition period which ends in July 2008 it will be compulsory for a dental nurse to be registered on the GDC's Dental Care Professionals Register, the only exception to this rule will be for trainee dental nurses, working under supervision and enrolled on a GDC-recognised course leading to Registration. There is currently no time limit on how long a dental nurse can work as a trainee. However, if they are unable to provide evidence of valid and current enrolment on a course then they cannot be counted as a trainee. You will only be able to work as unregistered until July 2008. The GDC will not accept applications on the basis of experience after this date.

Application for registration

It is best to get your application in as early as possible, as the initial registration fee (£72) will cover you until July 2009. After 2009 you will need to renew your registration fee on an annual basis. Applicants will need to provide:

- original qualifying certificate;
- statement of eligibility – for those entering through experience and the access to registration route;
- character reference – either a director of training or an employer or a professional peer who has known the applicant for minimum of two years;
- fitness to practise – evidence of good health.

Checks will be made on each applicant

- Criminal Record Bureau.
- Criminal convictions will be considered on a case by case basis.

With effect from July 2008, anyone using the title Dental Nurse whose name does not appear on the current DCP register could be prosecuted, unless they are enrolled on a recognised training programme.

Routes to registration for dental nurses open until July 2008
There will be one register for all groups of DCPs. Any dental nurse wishing to go on the DCP register will need to follow one of the following routes:

- Hold a registerable qualification, e.g. National Examining Board for Dental Nurses (NEBDN) National Certificate or NVQ/SVQ level 3 in Oral Healthcare – Dental Nursing.
- Membership of the National Voluntary Register for dental nurses.
- Four years' experience in the past eight years (full time or part time equivalent).
- Between two and four years' experience in the past eight years plus:

either
a statement of eligibility (from someone already registered who has personal knowledge of the applicant) certifying that they are competent in all six areas covered by the Access to Registration Training (ART) syllabus. The six areas are: cross-infection control; cardiopulmonary resuscitation and medical emergencies; health

and safety; ionising radiation; working with dentists and patients; and continuing professional development (CPD);
or
satisfactory completion of an ART course will include all six areas but will also need to be supported by a statement of eligibility (from someone already registered who has personal knowledge of the applicant) confirming that the applicant possesses the necessary skills and ability covered in the six areas plus a certificate, e.g. satisfactory completion of a GDC-approved ART course;
or
holds a certificate of satisfactory completion of ART in all six areas or holds a certificate which shows that the applicant has passed a GDC-approved Access to Registration Assessment (ARA). The assessment will be offered by NEBDN on a 'turn up and take basis'.

Indemnity cover – protecting your registration
The GDC has indicated that DCPs who advise or treat patients must ensure that they are indemnified against claims for professional negligence. Having professional indemnity cover means that the cost of any legal claims against you or threatened against you in the course of your professional work will be paid, plus the help and advice from a dento-legal advisor. It can also protect you against any personal liability for mishaps at work involving a patient (such as dropping an instrument on the patient).

You may think that this does not affect you and that you will be protected by your employer's liability policy. However, the GDC will take the view that it is your responsibility to check that the policy is sufficient to cover you fully. If you decide not to have professional indemnity cover you must be aware that you are accepting a risk that you will never become involved in a patient complaint, a disciplinary investigation or even a criminal investigation. In the event of a patient making a complaint to the GDC say, for example, concerning the standards of hygiene and sterilisation of instruments, it could be proved that the dental nurse was aware of the shortcomings and did not take appropriate action, In that case allegations could be made against the dental nurse. As a registered dental nurse you accept the responsibility as a dental professional, and cannot ignore things, particularly if patients are at risk. Realistically the chance of a claim for negligence being made against you by a patient or a lawyer is quite low, but certainly not impossible. A number of organisations offer professional indemnity for dental nurses (see Table 18.2 below for details).

Working in a team (Figure 18.1)
Working in a first-rate team can lead to a stress-free environment and is crucial for successful delivery of quality patient-centred care. There has been much written and said about teamwork, it seems at last that the benefits are being recognised and implemented. The GDC has produced a useful guidance document entitled *Principles of Dental Team Working*.

Working in a team means that individuals are valued and feel able to contribute to the organisation and smooth running of the surgery and have their views heard and respected. The team leader (not necessarily the dentist) will need to make sure that the strategic objectives of the practice are understood and that everyone is involved and committed to the plans.

The dentist's role is to be responsible for diagnosis, treatment planning and quality control of the treatment provided. A good leader will:

- have a strong customer focus – a patient-centred approach;
- be obsessive about providing quality dentistry;
- understand the role and value of each team member;
- develop and motivate the team through continuing education and training;
- look for faults and take responsibility for the professional conduct of the team ensuring that the patient is protected at all times;
- involve all team members in regular meetings to consult, agree and update everyone on new systems and procedures ensuring their co-operation.

18

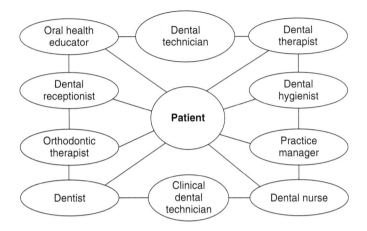

Fig. 18.1 The patient-centred team.

We can't all be the team leader, and other roles within the team are equally important. Your skills may be:

- supervising and urging the team to fulfil their roles and get on with the task in hand;
- easing tension and maintaining harmonious working relationships;
- producing carefully considered plans and improving on the ideas of others.

Whatever your skills may be you are an important member of the team, without you the team would not function as effectively.

Investors in People is a useful tool for teams wanting to identify themselves as a successful organisation. Many dental practices are achieving this nationally recognised standard. Working in an environment where teamwork operates well could reduce some of the stresses experienced during your working life.

Not all members of the team will be subject to statutory registration; this does not mean that their role within the team is any less valuable.

Dental receptionists

The role of the dental receptionist is crucial to the success of a dental practice as they represent the practice as the first impression for the patient. A number of training programmes are available and they have their own professional association (see Table 18.2 for details). A receptionist's role includes:

- front of house – meet and greet patients and callers – running the appointments system;
- promoting and marketing the practice and services;
- taking payments – answering telephone enquiries – retrieving and storing patient records;
- registering patients.

Practice managers

Practice managers do not necessarily have a dental background, many hold general management qualifications. Some are experienced dental nurses who have chosen to specialise in practice management. The professional association can advise about training programmes (see Table 18.2 for details). The Practice Manager's role includes: leading on the business planning; staff recruitment and management; planning future development for the practice; ordering and payment of invoices for stock items; financial management budgets and accounts.

Dental care professionals

This title was introduced in 2005 and includes team members who were previously called professionals complementary to dentistry. From 2006 all the following groups of professionals will be required to register with the GDC on the DCP Register:

- dental nurses;
- dental technicians;
- dental hygienists;
- dental therapists;
- clinical dental technicians;
- orthodontic therapists.

18

Scope of practice

The permitted duties of each DCP group will be managed through a system of regulation via curricula and ethical guidance. In 2004 a GDC document was published which detailed the areas of competence, knowledge and understanding required for each DCP group, it will be important for dental nurses to be familiar with this document – *Developing the Dental Team – Curricula Frameworks for Registerable Qualifications for PCDs* (2004). Under the terms of statutory registration dental nurses will have to limit their activity to the tasks in which they have trained and are competent. The GDC curricula framework is organised so that there is a section which is common and relevant to training programmes for all DCPs; it includes knowledge and understanding, skills and attitudes.

The GDC guidance suggests a minimum training period of 45 weeks (full time or part time equivalent) for a dental nurse. Here are a few examples of subjects and topics in the **dental nursing curriculum**; some will be familiar and expected but there may be some new things to learn.

- **Chairside support** – be able to demonstrate consistent practical ability and have knowledge of the clinical procedures associated with:
  –assessment of oral health;
  –treatment planning;
  –restorative dentistry;
  –paediatric dentistry;
  –orthodontics;
  –preventive dentistry;
  –oral surgery;
  –oral medicine;
  –gerodontology;
  –pain and anxiety control;
  –dental accidents and emergency dental care.
- **Behavioural sciences, communication skills and health informatics**
  –be competent in using information technology; communicating with patients, their families, and other team members and other health care professionals;

–have knowledge of managing patients from different social and ethnic backgrounds, working in a dental team.

- **Law, ethics and professionalism**
  - –be competent at maintaining full accurate records;
  - –have knowledge of responsibilities of consent, duty of care and confidentiality, patients' rights and how to handle complaints, the competency range of other members of the team, regulatory function of the GDC;
  - –be familiar with legal and ethical obligations of registered members of the dental team; the obligation to practise in the best interests of the patient at all times; the need for lifelong learning and professional development; and the law as it applies to records.

The full details of this document can be found on the GDC website (www.gdc-uk.org.uk).

An update on the competencies of other DCP team members

If we are to be recognised as members of the team we need to understand the roles and areas of competence of our DCP colleagues as well as our own. The scope of practice changes from time to time, the introduction of new professional groups such as clinical dental technicians and orthodontic therapists will be challenging but will offer more career options for dental nurses.

Dental technician

Dental technicians are the second largest DCP group (dental nurses are the largest), their role is to design, prepare and manufacture individual custom-made dental devices. They work independently to a dentist or doctor's prescription; there are three areas of expertise covered in their training (minimum training period 120 weeks – full time or part time equivalent). Below is an example of some of the competencies relating to dental technology. A dental technician should be competent in one of these areas:

- fixed prosthodontics;
- removable prosthodontics;
- orthodontics.

This includes:

- crown and bridgework construction: inlays, crowns and bridges in metal and ceramic/polymeric materials;
- prosthetics – designing and manufacturing complete dentures with polymeric bases, removable partial dentures with cast metal, framework or polymeric bases, occlusal splints;
- orthodontics – designing and manufacturing removable appliances and their modification and repair.

Dental hygienists and dental therapists

The training of hygienists and therapists is now often combined and the future may bring further integration with the roles eventually merging into one. The minimum training period for dental hygienists is 90 weeks. The dental therapist course requires an additional 12 weeks on top of the hygiene training (102 weeks altogether (full time)). Hygienists and therapists work in dental hospitals, community service and general dental practice. Below are examples of areas in which dental hygienists should be competent.

- Screening and monitoring dental diseases: instructing patients in methods of plaque control; instructing patients in the methods of preventing caries, dietary advice and the use of fluoride; checking and evaluating a patient's medical history and treatment plan, administration of local infiltration and inferior dental block analgesia; supra and subgingival scaling, root debridement, removal of stain and prophylaxis – the application of fissure sealants; use of topical fluoride; providing smoking cessation advice to patients.
- In addition to the above a dental therapist should be competent in the following areas, provided a registered dentist has examined the patient and indicated in writing the treatment plan to be followed by the therapist: placement of temporary dressings, temporary cementation of crowns and taking impressions; placement of amalgam and tooth coloured restorations in both permanent and deciduous teeth; extraction of deciduous teeth under local analgesia.

- Taking and processing dental radiographs used in general dental practice.

Clinical dental technician

There are currently no training programmes available in the UK. However there is training available in Canada and the Netherlands. Plans are under way to introduce a Diploma in Clinical Dental Technology in the first instance for dental technicians already holding the George Brown College Canadian qualification. The GDC guidance suggests a minimum of 90 weeks full time or part time training. Clinical dental technicians will be able to work independently.

The GDC curriculum for clinical dental technicians describes the areas of competence. These include:

- obtaining a relevant medical history;
- undertaking a clinical examination and following a treatment plan;
- taking and processing dental radiographs related to the provision of removable dental appliances;
- provision, repair and refurbishment of removable dental appliances, e.g. complete and removable partial dentures, mouth guards, retainers and splints but excluding orthodontic appliances.

Orthodontic therapist

Plans are under way to introduce a new qualification. It is likely that a dental nurse will see this as a natural progression, especially the one holding the NEBDN Certificate in Orthodontic Nursing and who has already covered much of the theoretical aspects of the training.

It will be necessary for a person entering orthodontic therapy training to be already qualified and registered in dental nursing, dental hygiene, dental therapy or dental technology, and have at least one year's post qualification experience. The GDC guidance suggests that a minimum period of training should be 45 weeks full time or part time equivalent. The GDC curriculum for orthodontic therapists describes the areas of competence. These include:

- taking intra-oral and extra-oral photographs;
- taking impressions;
- casting and trimming models;
- taking and checking occlusal records;
- producing cephalometric analyses of skull radiographs;
- inserting passive and active removable appliances, fitting orthodontic headgear (previously adjusted by a dentist);
- cleaning and preparing the tooth surface for orthodontic bonding;
- placing and removing orthodontic separators – placing, adapting and cementing bands;
- inserting and ligating archwires;
- releasing and removing ligatures and removing archwires;
- removing cemented and bonded attachments;
- removing orthodontic adhesive and cement residues from the teeth;
- supragingival cleaning;
- polishing and stain removal of teeth where directly relevant to orthodontic treatment.

CAREER PROGRESSION

As a registered dental nurse you have options and opportunities available should you wish to make a change in your working situation. Here are some career histories of dental nurses showing their chosen career paths. Perhaps you will recognise some similarity with your own experience so far.

Jill (Figure 18.2)

Jill works in a general dental practice in Manchester where she is the head dental nurse in charge of six dental nurses – four qualified and two in training. Jill has been working at the practice for eight years. She lives with her daughter and works flexible hours so that she can spend time with her. Jill started her dental nursing career as a youth trainee working at the dental hospital; she passed her national exam and went on to work in the department of restorative dentistry. While at the hospital she took the opportunity to study for the Certificate in Oral Health and passed

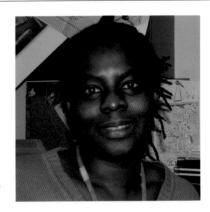

Fig. 18.2 Jill – Head dental nurse in general dental practice.

having completed her portfolio and passed the written examination.

Jill was keen to use her new qualification and decided to apply for a post in general dental practice. The advertisement said that the practice wanted to develop an oral health unit within the practice. Having the Oral Health Certificate helped Jill gain the position and she enjoyed designing and planning the new area which is a dedicated space for trained dental nurses to advise patients on how to improve their oral health. The dentists were very pleased with the success of the new unit, which is now a busy area within the practice. As a result Jill was given a good pay increase to reward her for her efforts. Since then Jill has completed the Radiography Certificate and is now responsible for taking most of the X-rays in the practice. Jill has always been supported and encouraged by the practice team and she feels that she is able to progress within the practice and hopes to continue working there.

Beverley (Figure 18.3)
Beverley is a dental nurse training manager. She has established herself in this senior position at a dental hospital in London where she lives with her husband and two children. Beverley has been an active member of the British Association of Dental Nurses

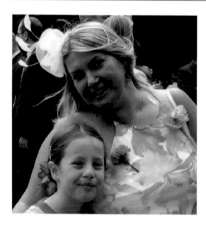

Fig. 18.3 Beverley – Dental nurse training manager with her daughter.

and the National Examining Board for Dental Nurses. Being involved with these professional bodies has helped Beverley to be well informed and up to date with current training issues, and be successful in her career.

Beverley worked her way up within the organisation where she started as a dental nurse student. Once qualified she worked with a consultant in the children's department where she was able to gain experience working in a dental theatre. Although she enjoyed working with children she knew that she wanted to be a tutor so she joined a course leading to the Further Adult Education Teaching Certificate at a local college. At around the same time Beverley was appointed as senior dental nurse and she gained new management skills and experience of being responsible for 12 qualified dental nurses and four student dental nurses. After a few years and having achieved her teaching qualification Beverley was successful in achieving her goal and became a tutor with the dental nursing school. That was over 10 years ago and Beverley is still learning new skills and meeting new challenges. Beverley is currently studying for a Masters degree in Educational Management which she hopes will enhance her position.

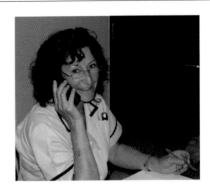

Fig. 18.4 Anita – Senior dental nurse in a district general hospital.

Anita (Figure 18.4)

Anita works as a senior dental nurse at a district general hospital in Yorkshire. She is responsible for the dental nurses in the orthodontic unit and manages the day-to-day activity. Anita has been a dental nurse for 15 years. Before that she had worked in a bank for six years. A friend who worked at the hospital suggested that she apply for a vacant post as a dental receptionist in the orthodontic unit. Anita's application was successful and she found the orthodontic work fascinating, so much so that she decided to start dental nurse training at her local College of Further Education. The evening classes were quite tough as she had no experience, but she had lots of help from the dental nurses in the unit. Anita was offered a training post within the unit and once she had passed the National Certificate was appointed as a qualified dental nurse. After a few years Anita had gained confidence and experience; she found the work rewarding and the staff friendly. Anita was still only earning the same pay as she received working in the bank! Fortunately a vacancy for a senior dental nurse came up and she was interviewed and appointed. The pay increase helped her to buy a computer and the books she needed to do the orthodontic nursing qualification which she has just started. She hopes that one day she will be able to work as an orthodontic therapist.

Continuing professional development

Just like dentists DCPs will be required to undertake continuing professional development (CPD). This is likely to become compulsory at the end of the transitional period when dental nurse and dental technician registration is compulsory. The GDC introduced continuing professional development for dentists to promote high standards and to ensure the protection of the public.

Patients can be sure that their dentist and DCPs are keeping up to date and are constantly acquiring new knowledge and skills. At present we are not aware what the exact requirements for DCPs will be, but it is likely to be similar to the requirements for current registrants. Below are details of those requirements.

Requirements for CPD for current registrants in order to remain on the register:

- 250 hours regular and frequent CPD over a five-year cycle – this includes part time and retired registrants;
- 75 hours of verifiable CPD – usually certificated and approved;
- submit an annual statement of hours to the GDC.

How will dental nurses benefit from CPD?

Apart from being a statutory requirement, you will probably be aware of your own strengths and weaknesses and be able to direct your CPD towards the areas where you need to improve or have a special interest for future career development.

It is important to have this in mind when you are preparing for a job interview so that you can judge whether you will be given the opportunities you need in order to progress. When you have an appraisal with your manager you will be able to ensure that, when discussing your appraisal objectives, they are in line with your needs as well as the needs of your employer. When you are starting out in your career it is often difficult to recognise your strengths and weaknesses. There may be someone at work or a good friend who could help you and act as a mentor. A mentor is someone you respect who has your interests at heart

Task 1 – Tick which skills are involved in your job role.

Task 2 – When you have identified the above, tick the skills you need to develop on the grid below.

SKILLS ANALYSIS					
SKILLS	**TASK 1**	**TASK 2**	**SKILLS**	**TASK 1**	**TASK 2**
Working with numbers			Helping others		
Working with others			Listening		
Managing money			Taking responsibility		
Finding out			Drive and initiative		
Interpreting data			Working under pressure		
Providing information			Analysing		
Leading a group			Being creative		
Working alone			Tact and sensitivity		
Discussing			Writing instructions		
Communicating			Following instructions		
Solving problems			Explaining things		
Understanding others			Supervising others		
Planning			Researching		
Diagnosing			Dealing with problems		
Making decisions			Organising events		
Having good ideas			Timekeeping		
Organising things			Taking risks		
Organising people			Persuading		

Fig. 18.5 Skills analysis.

and understands the dental scene; your conversations can be frank and open and always confidential. If you cannot identify a mentor at present then you should try using self-review. Use the skills analysis sheet (Figure 18.5) to identify existing skills and those you need to develop.

Make some decisions about what you want to achieve in your work within the next 12 months.

Record as many goals as you want and say why you want to achieve them.

When you have listed all of your goals determine a priority goal.

What I want to achieve (my goals)	Why I want to achieve these goals
(1)	
(2)	
(3)	
(4)	
(5)	
(6)	
(7)	
(8)	
(9)	
(10)	
My priority goal at the moment	

Fig. 18.6 Goals for the next 12 months.

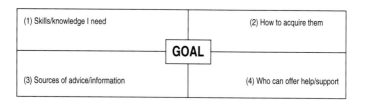

Fig. 18.7 Developing skills and knowledge.

Figure 18.6 can be used to help you identify your goals and Figure 18.7 will assist in planning how to develop your knowledge and skills in order to achieve your priority goal. Keep a record of your completed reviews in your personal folder so that you can reflect on them when you repeat the exercise (at least once a year).

Some ideas for your CPD:

- reading articles in professional journals;
- watching a DVD or dental programme;
- attending a meeting of a dental professional organisation;
- attending a short course;
- completing a formal training leading to a qualification.

Keeping a personal record (Figure 18.8)

As the GDC will require an annual statement of your CPD hours it would be helpful to keep a personal CPD log of your activities. Below are examples of items to be recorded and retained in the log.

Suggested contents of a Personal Continuing Professional Development log (*indicates the requirements of the GDC)

- Name*
- Period covered from . . . to . . .
- Title of event – activity*

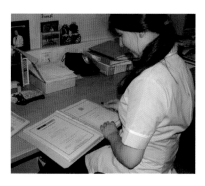

Fig. 18.8 Keeping up to date with CPD records.

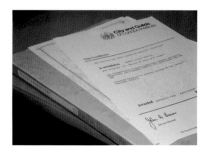

Fig. 18.9 A personal development folder.

- Dates attended*
- Hours undertaken*
- Venues*
- Training/provider*
- Key learning outcomes
- Relevance to your role
- Evidence reference – verifiable certificates*
- Comments*

Personal development folder/career portfolio
This is another useful record to have and keep up to date. As you gain more experience you will need to have a personal portfolio which will act as a permanent reference to help when:

- applying for further training and education;
- completing an application form;
- reviewing your progress.

Ideas for inclusion in your portfolio (Figure 18.9)
- Up-to-date curriculum vitae – this document usually includes details of:
  –personal;
  –training and education;
  –qualifications;
  –working experience;

–current position;
–personal achievements;
–membership of professional bodies;
–published work.
- original certificates – qualifications and courses attended;
- current and previous job descriptions;
- registration certificate and number;
- membership details of professional organisations/trade unions;
- contract of employment;
- annual appraisal objectives;

The Golden Rules

(1) The patient comes first – not your employer.

(2) If the patient knows what they want do your best to ensure they get it.

(3) The Senior Dental Nurse/Practice Manager is usually right – respect his/her opinion.

(4) Be kind to yourself – you are not inexhaustible.

(5) Give the patient (and yourself) time: time to ask questions and time to reflect.

Reflective practice

There is enormous benefit to be gained by stopping to reflect. It is far too easy to ignore your niggling doubts about an issue and tell yourself that you are too busy to stop and think. You owe yourself the time to ask – am I making the best of my skills and opportunities? Why not make a commitment to reflect on your situation at least once a year (maybe your birthday would be a good time).

Try writing down your strengths and weaknesses and consider whether you could improve your working life, you may also find this improves your personal lifestyle as well. Keeping up to date is important and meeting colleagues at meetings is a good way to ensure that you are informed about local and national issues. Most professional organisations have a journal or newsletter which will provide current information on dental topics and tell you about meetings in your area (please see Tables 18.1 and 18.2 for details of professional organisations).

The conclusions you reach following a period of reflection will also help to identify issues you wish to raise at your next appraisal with your manager. You may decide to that you want to change your hours of work or study for a new qualification or even change your career.

Fig. 18.10 The Golden Rules.

- references;
- relevant correspondence;
- copies of any published works, etc.

Post-certification qualifications

For those who want to specialise in a particular aspect of dental nursing a number of options are available, and there will be more to come as dental nurses expand their duties. This outlines the main qualifications. The usual entry requirement is that the dental nurse is registered and has the agreement of a dentist to act as a supervisor. Please see Table 18.1 below for further information. Figure 18.10 shows a few Golden Rules to help you improve your working life.

Table 18.1 Awarding body information

Awarding body	Details of the qualification
National Examining Board for Dental Nurses www.nebdn.org.uk	**Certificate in Oral Health Education** Suitable for qualified dental nurses who intend to give oral health advice to patients either on a one-to-one basis or in small groups – would be helpful for those wishing to train as a dental hygienist/therapist
National Examining Board for Dental Nurses www.nebdn.org.uk	**Certificate in Orthodontic Nursing** Suitable for qualified dental nurses who assist in orthodontic procedures – would be helpful for those wishing to train as an orthodontic therapist
National Examining Board for Dental Nurses www.nebdn.org.uk	**Certificate in Dental Radiography** Suitable for qualified dental nurses who may act as an operator under the Ionising Radiation (Medical Exposure) Regulations – this is a qualification which is useful for all dental care professorials
National Examining Board for Dental Nurses www.nebdn.org.uk	**Certificate in Dental Sedation Nursing** Suitable for qualified dental nurses who assist in the surgery during routine conscious sedation – you need to be working in this area in order to complete the portfolio of experience which is part of the qualification
National Examining Board for Dental Nurses www.nebdn.org.uk	**Certificate in Special Care Dentistry** Suitable for qualified dental nurses who assist during the treatment of people whose health and social care needs may require special oral healthcare provision – this qualification is popular with dental nurses working in the community service

Continued

Table 18.1 *Continued*

British Dental Practice Managers Association www.bdpma.org.uk (not an Awarding Body but a good source of information about training providers and locations) www.bdpma.org.uk	Diploma in Management Level 4 (Institute of Leadership and Management) Executive Diploma in Management Level 5 (Institute of Leadership and Management) Edexel Certificates and Diploma in Management in Level 3, 4 and 5
City & Guilds www.city-and-guilds.org.uk These qualifications are also offered by other awarding bodies	**Assessor Award** A short course suitable for qualified dental nurses who are involved in the assessment of trainees completing an NVQ programme
City & Guilds www.city-and-guilds.org.uk	**Internal Verifiers Award (V1)** A short course suitable for qualified dental nurses who are training to become internal verifiers carrying out a quality assurance process of NVQ Awards
Chartered Institute of Environmental Health www.cieh.org	**Foundation Award in Health and Safety in the Workplace** A short course for those who want to increase their knowledge and gain better understanding of health and safety in the workplace
Chartered Institute of Environmental Health www.cieh.org	**Risk Assessment Principles and Practice Certificate** Suitable for dental nurses who carry out risk assessments, under the management of the Health and Safety at Work Regulations 1999

18

Table 18.2 Useful contact details

(A) Professional organisations for dental nurses	Resources available to members
British Association of Dental Nurses Hillhouse International Business Centre Thornton, Cleveleys, Lancashire FY5 4QD Tel 01253 338360 www.badn.org.uk	Journal 'The British Dental Nurse' National Representation – advice Regional Groups Special interest sub-groups, e.g. **National Teaching Group** Orthodontics – Special care and sedation dental nursing
Orthodontic National Group Affiliated to the British Orthodontic Society 11, Woodberry Close Chiddingfold, Surrey GU8 4SF Tel 01428 684855 www.orthodontic-ong.co.uk	Newsletter Conferences Advice Study days
National Examining Board for Dental Nurses 108–110 London Street Fleetwood, Lancashire FY7 6EU Tel 01253 778417 www.nebdn.org.uk	Qualifications and advice on training provision National Certificate – N/SVQ Oral Health Certificate Orthodontics – Radiography Sedation – Special Care
Faculty of General Dental Practitioners (UK) Dental Care Professional Affiliate Membership The Royal College of Surgeons of England 35–43 Lincoln's Inn Fields London WC2A 3PE Tel 020 7869 6754 www.fgdp.org.uk	Journal 'Team in Practice' DCP Advisory Board Team-based education Local divisions Continuing Professional Development courses
Amicus Hayes Court, West Common Road Hayes, Bromley, Kent BR2 7AU Tel 0845 850 4242 www.amicustheunion.org	Trade union for people delivering public services – includes hospital and community services Campaigns and lobbies on key issues affecting its members
Unison 1 Mableton Place London WC1 9AJ Tel 0845 355 0845 www.unison.org.uk	Trade Union for people delivering public services – includes hospital and community services Campaigns and lobbies on key issues affecting its members
(B) Governing bodies	
General Dental Council 37 Wimpole Street London W1G 8DQ Tel 020 7887 3800 www.gdc-uk.org	Information all aspects Registration – guidance documents Maintaining Standards Education Patient Leaflets Gazette

Continued

Table 18.2 *Continued*

Department of Health	Policy documents
79 Whitehall	Guidance notes
London	Statistics
SW1A 2NS	Consultation
020 72104850	Publications
www.doh.gov.uk	

(C) Other DCP associations — **Resources available to members**

British Dental Receptionists' Association	Newsletter
24, Farnworth Grove	Advice on training
Birmingham	Conferences
B36 9JA	National representation
Tel 0870 0801924	
www.bdra.co.uk	
British Dental Practice Managers	Training
Osprey House, Primett Road	Advice sheets
Stevenage, Herts	Regional seminars
SG1 3EE	Conference
Tel 0870 84000381	
www.bdpma.org.uk	
British Dental Hygienists' Association	Journal
Mobbs Miller House, Ardington Road	Conference
Northampton	National representation
NN1 5LP	Advice
Tel 0870 2430752	Regional meetings
www.bdha.org.uk	
British Association of Dental Therapists	Training school information
75 Millfield Parc, Newport Road	Events and courses
Magor	Annual scientific meeting
NP2 63LL	
Dental Technicians' Association	Careers in dental technology
PO Box 6520	
Northampton	
NN3 9ZX	
www.dta-uk.org	
Clinical Dental Technician Association	About clinical dental
12 Upper Street North	technology
New Ash Green, Kent	
DA3 8JR	
Tel 01474 879430	
www.cdta.org.uk	

(D) Other useful contacts

British Dental Health Foundation	Supports dental professionals
Smile House	by providing information,
2 East Union Street	resources for oral health
Rugby	education and promotion
CV22 6JA	
Tel 0845 0603	
www.dentalhealth.org.uk	

18

Continued

Table 18.2 *Continued*

British Fluoridation Society Ward 4 Booth Hall Children's Hospital Charlestown Road Blackley, Manchester M9 7AA Tel 0161 2205223 www.bfsweb.org	Aims to improve the dental health of the UK population by the implementation of the government's policy on water fluoridation
NHS Business Services Authority – Dental Practice Division (formerly Dental Practice Board for England & Wales) Compton Place Road Eastbourne, East Sussex BN20 8AD Tel 01323 433550 www.dpb.nhs.uk	Support DOH in determining policy and strategy – produces statistics and key information Transfers payment to dentists Publications Help desk
Health and Safety Executive (See website for local offices) www.hsedirect.com	Government agency which aims to ensure that risk to people's health and safety from workplace activities are properly controlled Help line – publications
National Institute for Health and Clinical Excellence (NICE) MidCity Place, 71 High Holborn London WC1V 6NA Tel 020 7067 5800 www.nice.org.uk	Independent organisation responsible for providing national guidance and promoting good health and preventing and treating ill health
Investors in People (IiP) 7–10 Chandos Street London W1G 9DQ Tel 020 7467 1900 www.investorinpeople.co.uk	The IiP standard is a widely recognised business improvement tool. Designed to advance an organisation's performance through its people
Dental Protection Ltd 33 Cavendish Square London W1G OPS Tel 020 7399 1400 www.dentalprotection.org.uk	Professional indemnity insurance Provides support, advice and assistance in all matters that challenge the integrity of dental professionals
Medical and Dental Defence Union of Scotland Mackintosh House 120 Blythswood Street Glasgow G2 4EA Tel 0141 221 5858 www.mddus.com	Professional indemnity insurance Provides advice and support
The Dental Defence Union 230 Blackfriars Road London SE1 8PJ Tel 020 7202 1500 www.the-ddu.com	Professional indemnity insurance Advice – helpline Publications Information

18

REFERENCES

General Dental Council (2004) *Developing the Dental Team – Curricula Framework for Registerable Qualifications for Professionals Complementary to Dentistry.* London, General Dental Council.

General Dental Council guidance (2005) *Principles of Dental Team Working Standards for Dental Professionals.* London, General Dental Council.

Dental Materials and Equipment

DENTAL MATERIALS

All dental materials should be mixed and stored according to manufacturer's instructions, paying particular attention to mixing and setting times.

Zinc oxide and eugenol cement

Constituents
- Powder – zinc oxide.
- Liquid – eugenol.

Uses
Temporary dressing, lining in deep cavities.

Special properties
Sedative.

Zinc oxide and eugenol paste

Constituents
- Paste 1 – zinc oxide.
- Paste 2 – eugenol.

Uses
Impression material for complete dentures.

Zinc phosphate

Constituents
- Powder – zinc oxide and freeze-dried phosphoric acid.
- Liquid – distilled water.

Uses
Temporary filling, cavity lining, cementation of crowns, bridges, inlays and orthodontic bands.

Glass ionomer cement

Constituents
- Powder – aluminosilicates and freeze-dried polyacrylic acid.
- Liquid – distilled water.

Uses
Restorations (particularly cervical), cementation of crowns, bridges, etc.

Special properties
- Releases fluoride.
- Bonds directly to enamel and dentine.
- Can be etched.

Alginate

Constituents
- Powder.
- Liquid – room temperature water.

Uses
Impressions for study models, orthodontic appliances, dentures, etc.

Rubber-based impression material

Constituents
Vary from brand to brand.

Uses
Impressions for crowns, bridges, veneers, etc.

Polycarboxylate cement

Constituents
- Powder – zinc oxide and freeze-dried polyacrylic acid.
- Liquid – distilled water.

Uses
Cavity lining, cementation of crowns, bridges, etc.

Calcium hydroxide

Constituents
Two-paste system containing calcium hydroxide and a setting agent.

Uses
Cavity lining.

Special properties
Can promote the production of secondary dentine.

DENTAL INSTRUMENTS
A range of dental instruments have been introduced in the preceding chapters, however as handpieces and burs are used throughout clinical dentistry, they are included in this chapter.

Handpieces

High-speed handpiece (also known as air turbine handpiece)
These handpieces are used in conjunction with friction grip burs (see below) for cutting enamel (Figure 19.1).

Contra-angle handpiece
These handpieces are used in conjunction with latch grip burs (see below) usually for cutting dentine (Figure 19.2).

19

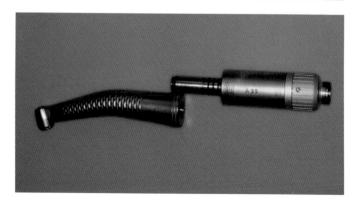

Fig. 19.1 High-speed handpiece with motor.

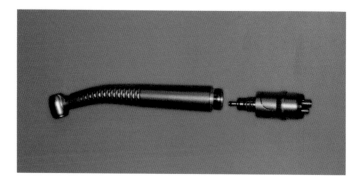

Fig. 19.2 Contra-angle handpiece.

Straight laboratory handpiece
Used when trimming dentures or orthodontic appliances in conjunction with long shank burs (see below) (Figure 19.3).

Surgical handpiece
Used when drilling bone during a surgical procedure. Usually has a saline drip attached. Surgical burs (see below) are used with this handpiece (Figure 19.4).

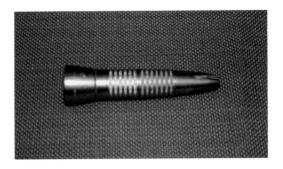

Fig. 19.3 Straight laboratory handpiece.

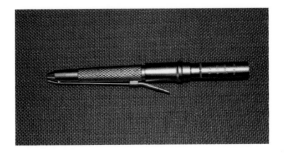

Fig. 19.4 Surgical handpiece.

Burs

Head shapes

Whatever a bur may be made from and whatever shank they may have, there are a range of shapes which apply to all burs (Figure 19.5).

So you may have a rosehead (round) green stone or a rosehead (round) stainless steel bur and although they look very different the head shape is the same.

19

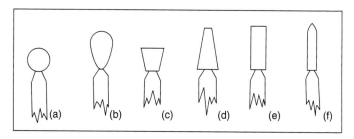

Fig. 19.5 Different shapes of bur heads. (a) Rosehead; (b) pear; (c) inverted cone; (d) tapered fissure; (e) flat fissure; (f) flame.

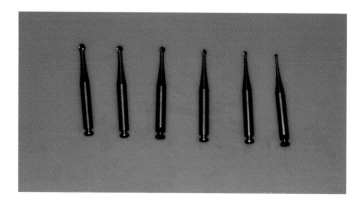

Fig. 19.6 Stainless steel burs.

19

Construction

Burs can be made from stainless steel, tungsten carbide, diamond, stone or rubber.

- **Stainless steel** burs are used, in conjunction with the contra-angle handpiece, for cutting dentine and polishing amalgam and are most often available with a latch grip shank (Figure 19.6). Burs used for cutting acrylic are also made from stain-

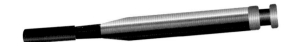

Fig. 19.7 Tungsten carbide bur.

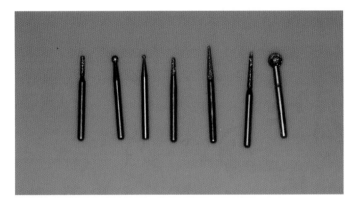

Fig. 19.8 Diamond burs.

less steel and are available with long shanks. These are used in a laboratory handpiece. Surgical burs are usually made from stainless steel too and have a surgical shank for use with a surgical handpiece.

- **Tungsten carbide** burs are distinctive by their head being darker than their shank and are usually used with the air turbine handpiece for cutting through enamel (Figure 19.7).
- **Diamond burs** are rough headed burs and are also used with the air turbine handpiece for cutting through enamel (Figure 19.8).
- **Stones** and **rubber** tipped burs are used for polishing and can be available either with a latch grip shank or a long shank (Figure 19.9).

19

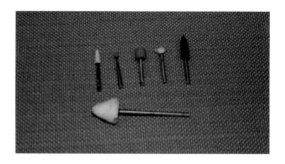

Fig. 19.9 Stones and rubber tipped burs.

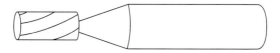

Fig. 19.10 Latch grip shank.

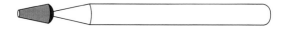

Fig. 19.11 Friction grip shank.

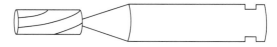

Fig. 19.12 Long shank.

Shanks
- Latch grip – for use with contra-angle handpiece (Figure 19.10).
- Friction grip – for use with air turbine handpiece (Figure 19.11).
- Long shank – for use with laboratory handpiece (Figure 19.12).

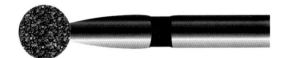

Fig. 19.13 Surgical shank.

• Surgical shank – for use with surgical handpiece (Figure 19.13).

Periodontal Treatment and Prevention of Dental Disease

Periodontal treatment can range from something as simple as a scale and polish to something as complex as periodontal surgery. The aim of periodontal treatment is to treat the effects of periodontal disease including gingivitis.

SCALE AND POLISH

(1) Prepare the surgery and seat the patient in the dental chair. Provide the patient and dental team with personal protective equipment.
(2) The dental nurse may be required to retract the soft tissues and aspirate while the operator removes calculus using scalers and curettes.
(3) A mouthwash may be offered to the patient at this stage.
(4) Prophylaxis paste is dispensed and handed to the operator who will polish the patient's teeth using a prophylaxis paste and either a prophy brush or a rubber cup.
(5) Again the dental nurse may offer the patient a mouthwash and assist them with cleaning their face.
(6) Oral health instructions may be given to the patient by the dental nurse (see below).

GINGIVECTOMY

Gingivectomy is an oral surgery procedure (see Chapter 7) carried out to remove excess gingival tissue to create a new gingival margin. It is carried out when gingivitis does not respond to treatment and strict oral hygiene procedures.

(1) Once the patient is prepared for surgery the dental nurse will retract the soft tissue and aspirate as the gingiva is trimmed by the operator.

(2) If sutures are required the dental nurse may assist with this process by cutting the sutures as directed by the operator.

(3) A periodontal pack may also be applied to protect the area and the dental nurse can assist by applying Vaseline (petroleum jelly) around the patient's mouth and mixing the material ready for use.

(4) Post-operative instructions (see below) can be given by the dental nurse both orally and in writing.

POST-OPERATIVE INSTRUCTIONS

- **Painkillers** – it is difficult to predict the degree of discomfort that will be experienced. Usually it is tolerable but not always. Some painkillers may need to be provided for the journey home as the anaesthetic wears off.
- **Sutures** – there may be some stitches keeping the flaps in place around the teeth. Under no circumstances should these be removed at home. This will be done at the next appointment.
- **Packs** – a special pink pack may have been placed over the surgery site to keep the tissue in place. This should not be removed by the patient. If bleeding occurs this can be arrested by applying steady pressure to the area with a moist handkerchief or gauze for 30 minutes. It does not matter if part or all of the pack is lost.
- **Toothbrushes** – should the patient be brushing, flossing and bottle brushing? Yes but not the teeth involved in the surgery during the first week unless told to do so by the dentist.
- **Mouth-rinsing** – after 24 hours a hot salt water mouth wash should be used every four to six hours. Place a half teaspoonful of table salt in a tumbler of water as hot as can comfortably be held in the mouth. Gently and slowly rinse. This should give considerable relief.
- **Chlorhexidine mouth wash (Corsodyl)** – a bottle or prescription for a special mouth wash may have to be given. It is important to use this for the next two weeks **after** brushing at night and in the morning. Some staining may occur but this can be removed by the dentist at a later date.

- **Diet –** it would be wise to adopt a softer diet in the earlier stages and also to avoid hot or cold food and drink during the first 24 hours.
- **Daily routine** – exertion should be avoided in the first few days and a sensibly lighter schedule should be arranged in one's diary for the first 48 hours following the surgery.
- **Swelling** – some swelling may occur. This usually starts to subside after 48 hours.
- **Doubt** – if there are any concerns that healing is not going well the department should be contacted for appropriate advice. Smokers should quit for at least a week as smoking is known to cause problems with healing.

PREVENTION

Dental disease can be prevented by:

- good oral hygiene practices;
- healthy diet;
- regular dental visits;
- fissure sealants.

ORAL HEALTH ADVICE

- When giving oral health advice it is important to assess what the patient knows and is capable of before tailoring the advice to suit the individual.
- It may be helpful to use a disclosing solution as this will illustrate to the patient the need for good oral hygiene and identify the areas of most need.
- Techniques selected for the patient should be demonstrated using models and visual aids.
- The patient should then be asked to repeat the demonstration either on the model or on themselves to demonstrate understanding.
- Important information should be repeated to the patient and if necessary written down to reinforce the message.

20

ORAL HYGIENE MESSAGES

Toothbrushing
Toothbrushing advice should include the frequency of tooth-brushing, the type of toothbrush, the type of toothpaste and the method advised.

Floss
If advising the use of floss, the advice should include the type of floss recommended for use and the method for use.

Interproximal aids
A description of the interproximal aids available and the specific types recommended for use by the patient would be helpful as well as a demonstration of the method of use.

Mouthwashes
If a mouthwash is advised for the patient, ensure you are specific about the mouthwash required and the frequency and method of use.

DIETARY ADVICE
Patients should be advised of the effects of refined carbohydrates (sugars) on their teeth and where necessary should be asked to complete a diet diary prior to advice being given. This will enable the dental nurse to assess what the areas for concern are on an individual basis.

It may be necessary for the patient to be advised on the frequency of their sugar intake, preferably confining intake to meal times.

Foods containing hidden sugars may also need to be explained to the patient as well as sugar-free alternatives. It is important that the advice is tailored to the patient and reasonable achievable targets are set for improvement.

Index